Dear Kathy,

Sorry to hear about your illness. I'm glad you have your daughter Kristen to help you. I know it's tough as I'm a cancer patient, as well. I'll look for you on Facebook. I hope you enjoy this book. I'll be praying for you and thinking of you.

Fondly,

Mindy
Pete
Conquer

DEFY & CONQUER

PRAISE FOR DEFY & CONQUER

In this book, Mindy Elwell has chronicled her journey from brain tumor diagnosis, through her decision to use a ketogenic diet as an adjuvant therapy and its integration into her lifestyle...She includes detailed information, including hints and recipes [she has] discovered and created.

Defy & Conquer is an excellent resource for brain tumor patients... written from the point of view of a brain tumor patient and, therefore, providing information in a manner more suited to individuals dealing with the unique issues presented by this diagnosis.

Mindy not only provides insights from her own point of view but she also provides information about resources available to help empower brain tumor patients to pursue the use of this metabolic therapy in addition to the standard of care. We highly recommend this book for cancer patients interested in exploring the use of this diet as part of their treatment regimen.

Adrienne C. Scheck, Ph.D.
Associate Professor
Neuro-Oncology Research
Barrow Brain Tumor Research Center
Barrow Neurological Institute
Phoenix, AZ

Leonora Renda, RDN
University of Arizona Cancer Center
St. Joseph's Hospital and Medical Center
Phoenix, AZ

Mindy shares her powerful story with dignity and humor. Not even the insidious C-Club can stop her from soaking up every fierce, faithful, frightening moment of her beautiful life. Her story of strength and endurance serves as a reminder that life's fleeting moments are valuable treasures to be cherished. She shares her struggle with candor and wit. Although cancer patients and their caregivers will find valuable support and guidance in this book, readers from all walks of life will be impressed by Mindy's strength and humility.

Shelly Hornback
Arizona philanthropist and community leader

As a Patient Liaison at Barrow Neurological Institute, I often see patients that feel powerless when it comes to playing a part in both their treatment plan and the decision-making process. Mindy refused to give in to fear. Instead, she put together a team of incredible doctors, engaged whatever resources she could find, and educated herself, her team and her family. My own family has been touched by a very rare brain tumor (hypothalamic hamartoma) and I understand that sense of isolation, fear, and despair.

For me, taking control meant starting a nonprofit and educating others. For Mindy, it has been her amazing gift with words that has led her to create a book for everyone who has been touched not only by cancer but also by the many challenges of life. Through her faith, her positive attitude, and her willingness to expose the tender moments, she has shown us all that we can overcome the seemingly impossible. This book, and the life lessons it teaches, is a gift from a woman I admire greatly and am blessed to call a friend. I am thankful that she has shared her heart and her powerful story with us all.

Lisa Soeby
Patient Liaison, Barrow Neurological Institute
Co-founder, Hope for Hypothalamic Hamartomas

DEFY & CONQUER

Publisher's Disclaimer: Not all cancer patients will experience cancer the way Ms. Elwell did, nor will they respond the same to her treatment regimen or diet. If you are diagnosed with cancer, there is no more important source of information and guidance than your health professional. Defy & Conquer is not a replacement for professional medical care or advice, nor is it intended to be a How To in dealing with cancer. It is merely one brave woman's account against a deadly disease, shared with the public in the hopes of helping others cope and endure a similar situation.

Scripture (Matthew 6:25-34, 2 Corinthians 9) taken from *New King James Version*. Copyright © 1979, 1980, 1982 by Thomas Nelson, Inc. Used by permission. All rights reserved.

Hardcover   ISBN 978-1-939454-29-4
Softcover   ISBN 978-1-939454-30-0
Ebook   ISBN 978-1-939454-31-7
Library of Congress Control Number: 2015935828
Cataloging in Publication data pending.

Published in the United States by
Balcony 7 Media and Publishing
530 South Lake Avenue, Suite 434
Pasadena, CA 91101
www.balcony7.com

Cover and Book Design by 3 Dog Design

Printed in the United States of America

Distributed to the trade by
Ingram Publisher Services
Mackin
Overdrive
Baker & Taylor (through IPS)
MyiLibrary

DEFY
&
CONQUER

A STATE OF MIND AGAINST
TERMINAL BRAIN CANCER

MINDY ELWELL

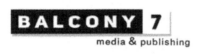
BALCONY 7
media & publishing

To Rich

my husband, best friend, protector, and

the love of my life

CONTENTS

Part II   The Ketogenic Diet, Supplements, Nutrition

FOREWORD

———

When I first met Mindy and Rich Elwell, they had just finished discussing the Ketogenic Diet with our wonderful registered dietitian Leonora Renda. They had asked to meet with me to hear about the research we've been doing regarding the use of the ketogenic diet for the treatment of malignant brain tumors. As I told them of our work and we chatted about how our results might apply to Mindy, I was struck by their upbeat, positive outlook and the excellent questions they asked. When Rich said he was going on the diet with Mindy, it was clear that, despite whatever challenges came up, these two were going to make this work.

The fact that metabolism in cancer cells is abnormal has been known since the 1920s, and we know that tumor cells don't use glucose for energy in the same way that normal cells do. While there have been some attempts to use this in the design of therapies, this was really not met with much enthusiasm, especially when molecular studies began to define genes involved in the formation of tumors.

There has been a recent resurgence in interest in the study of metabolism in cancer. In fact, alterations in metabolism are now considered a hallmark of cancer. This is underscored by the fact that many of the processes found to be involved in the formation of tumors actually intersect with processes involved in metabolism in cells. This suggests that therapies targeting metabolism may be effective for the treatment of cancers.

A caveat to this is that you can't simply reduce glucose and shut down metabolism without hurting normal cells. The high fat, low carbohydrate and protein ketogenic diet gets around this problem by providing ketones, which can be used by normal cells for energy. Cancer cells cannot use ketones—they require glucose.

The ketogenic diet has been used to treat epilepsy in people, particularly children, who don't respond to standard drugs. It has been shown to be safe. However, despite the long-standing safety record and mounting evidence in laboratory models showing utility of the ketogenic diet for the treatment of brain tumors, clinicians have been very slow to adopt this therapy.

It takes a strong individual and a supportive family to "go against the tide" and adopt a treatment that is not yet considered mainstream. Mindy and Rich chose to add the ketogenic diet to their fight against Mindy's tumor (Anaplastic Astrocytoma, Grade III), and in doing so they help to blaze a trail for other patients.

In this book, Mindy describes her journey in an intensely personal manner; however, it is done in a way that other brain tumor patients will be able to relate to. In addition, she shares insights she has gained along the way regarding how her diagnosis and the effects of the various therapies affected interactions with friends and family members. She has also shared information about how she has implemented the ketogenic dict. While the individual journey taken by cancer patients and their loved ones is unique, the knowledge that others have had many of the same thoughts and feelings can help one cope. This book will resonate with many cancer patients and give hope as they battle this devastating disease.

Adrienne C. Scheck, Ph.D.
Associate Professor, Neuro-Oncology Research
Barrow Brian Tumor Research Center
Barrow Neurological Institute
Phoenix, AZ

INTRODUCTION

When a doctor looks you in the eye and tells you a malignant tumor is growing in your brain, your world instantly changes. When I heard those words, I gasped. It was a reflexive reaction of pure disbelief. However, this tumor wasn't big enough to obstruct the whole of my life, my past and my lost future, from storming through my confused consciousness. Overwhelmed by it all, the rest of that day became a blur.

Immediately following my first MRI, I was catapulted into a whole new world of doctors, technicians, clinics and hospitals; blood tests, scans, radiation, medication, debilitation, side-effects, anxiety, fear—these replaced everything that was once my life. This rapid pace of events was necessary given the tumor's type and size. My family had no choice but to learn how to navigate this new, long and winding road, even though we weren't really sure what to expect. But we knew the two possible destinations: life or death. We steered toward life, in spite of the many detours and roadblocks we came across.

Everything became suddenly complex; there was so much to remember and so much to record. My husband and I started "the binder," which held everything regarding my treatment. Soon after, I started recording my own thoughts as well. I didn't know I would write a book until I realized, with as much certainty as God and my most recent MRI would grant me, that I might be beating this thing called cancer.

Cancer of any kind is unforgiving. A friend of mine who had colorectal cancer died as I was writing this. He fought hard and went through hell. My sympathy goes out to his wife and kids, his parents and siblings, and closest friends.

My feelings about what he went through are truly irrelevant, but what it's making clear in my life is the wonder of how much more time I have, what impact my life and existence may have on others. No, I'm not of the belief that my early death was predetermined for some bigger purpose. Even if some "good" were to come from me leaving Earth before a full lifespan, it's no easier for me to accept. But my story needs to be shared, maybe for just that reason.

I've outlived a bleak and short prognosis and it's important to pass on what I did to help others dealing with a brain tumor have a fighting chance. I include my nutritional regimen, my mental and physical health suggestions, links and lists for quick reference, along with my personal perspective and opinion to move an awful topic from misery to tolerance and, ultimately, to some advantage.

The newly diagnosed may benefit the most from reading my story, those who are feeling the raw disbelief and fear that follow a doctor's prognosis of possible death. But this book is also for all the others: survivors of brain cancer, those who have had brain surgery, caregivers, spouses, and—especially—the children of those touched by cancer's ominous reach. In my case, we have three children. Telling them they may lose their mother was heartbreaking. In this book, I share essays each of my kids wrote recounting what they felt after learning the news. Adults often say that kids are resilient, but they feel pain and their fears need to be addressed. I hope those of you with children may relate to what my family went through. We fought this together. That made me stronger, but it also made them stronger as well.

Writing about my two-year journey was not meant to be as much a "How-To" for someone in a similar position than to be a relatable guide. My intent was to describe what happened and outline my response to the biggest challenge I ever faced. The most important lesson I learned and wish to share is to be your own advocate. I took ownership of my disease and independently sought medical and nutritional counsel beyond the traditional cancer community. I questioned procedures and learned more about cancer than I could ever have possibly imagined. This knowledge quest was like a treasure hunt, leading me to additional kernels of hope. My husband and I didn't settle for living with this tumor, after a year of trying and it continuing to grow. It was too aggressive. We had to be even more aggressive.

We kept looking for that one doctor who would tell us, "Yes, we can do something about this. We can physically remove it from your body." That's what we wanted to hear. While this doesn't necessarily guarantee success, it gives hope. In the early stages, I lost hope. It was a lonely time, even though family surrounded me. I almost gave up; wished I would die in my sleep; contemplated suicide. All of that crossed my mind.

The personal space of someone touched by cancer remains intimately lonely. Despite the incessant publicity buzz surrounding cancer relays, races and fundraisers promoting awareness, the real peace that touches the cancer patient comes from within. Individual awareness, spirituality, mental strength, these are all very private tools no amount of money or research can offer. It certainly isn't easy to come by but I can sincerely say I've experienced more days of calm and enjoyment than tears; although the tears will come and aren't always controllable or predictable—nor are their triggers.

I offer a compilation of my experiences and reactions to a horrifying diagnosis, my path toward outliving my predicted demise, and what I've done to remain quite well up to this point. Through honest and candid descriptions of "a different kind of life," I hope you may relate and feel free to express your own fears and anxieties. Shedding that debilitating layer and moving forward unencumbered may allow you to see a different kind of "new normal;" with a vision made brighter by validation, empowerment and hope.

Throughout my writing I don't mince words or hold back. So many people I've talked to with a brain cancer diagnosis are extremely angry and entitled to be so. The sometimes angry and bitter thoughts that crossed my mind during my journey are illustrated colorfully here to give you permission to let yours out. State your opinion, own your situation and maximize what you've got. It's okay to say, "This is horrible and so very unfair." I'll help you fight like crazy. If I didn't, I'm quite sure I wouldn't have made it this long. As I said, I considered suicide. I wished for a heart attack so I would go quickly and quietly. I admit these terrible thoughts and I'm betting they're not uncommon.

It's important to note that everyone's experience will be unique, not necessarily like my own, which was deemed unusual by experts and care providers in the cancer community. Outliving my prognosis leaves me hopeful, content and comfortable. But in spite of differences in the individual journey, it doesn't hurt to mimic my approach: I busted out of the gate on warp speed, determined to be a Lone Ranger and to raise the bar on my goals. Undeterred optimism and faith wasn't always easy to come by but, when it was within my reach, I latched onto it for dear life. That's what helped me climb the steepest hills of my journey. I never stopped believing I could still enjoy a supreme life, even if it would be cut short, true to the doctors' predictions. This kind of attitude actually improved my quality of mind, which in turn improved my quality of life—no matter how long it would be. The time I had today became precious. Every day is, indeed, a gift.

If you are newly diagnosed, experiencing a recurrence, or caring for someone with brain cancer, I urge you to dig in, carry on, and fortify yourself with the knowledge that personal growth may, in fact, be obtained throughout this challenge. When faced with a life-changing moment involving terminal cancer, we have a choice. Rather than spend the rest of our days with bitterness, mentally surrendering our own life to an unseen enemy, we can capture any precious time we have and learn to appreciate it. With gratitude, grace, and a healthy dose of defiance, we may find salvation.

What keeps coming to the forefront of my thoughts are not wasting time on silly things and filling the air with words and complaints that don't add any quality to my existence or to the memories of my husband and kids. In the end, I'm going out alone. My kids and my husband will still have each other and will go on living their lives onward into the future. The thought of us being separated, however, brings me so much pain. Having been one of a pack of five for so long, it's just sickening to think of our family being anything but me (the eternally devoted mom), and Rich (the equally devoted husband and dad), with our three offspring, forever together.

Over the past two years, the greatest lesson I've learned is also the fiercest. I offer you this hard-earned thought:

Spiritual empowerment over cancer marks the moment we begin diminishing its power.

If you or a loved one is suffering from cancer, please join me. Together, we can defy and conquer.

TIMELINE OF EVENTS

2012

February	mid	First symptoms begin
	26	First MRI
March	3	Tumor board reviews my case
	7	MRI for neurological team
	8	Admitted to hospital for biopsy prep
	9	Brain tumor needle biopsy performed
	13	Discharged home; using a walker with difficulty; very fatigued; extreme sensitivity to noise & movement
	17	Begin physical therapy; difficulty walking
	25	Begin tests for treatment planning
April	1	Treatments are scheduled
	2	Radiation mask is fitted
	4	Radiation & daily oral chemotherapy begins
	6	Begin using a cane; still not walking well
	10	Started walking independently with cane
	16	Week 3 of treatments; able to exercise daily
	26	Hair falling out; tired, napping as needed; starting the Ketogenic Diet as adjuvant therapy

May	6	Week 5 complete; steadily improving
	17	Last day of radiation; 4-week break from chemo begins
June	15	First post-treatment MRI; allowed to drive again; results mixed
	25	Defining priorities; clear personal purpose forming
July	11	My 45th birthday; enhanced MRI reading shows, "It's not great news but not terrible...;"
August	13	Labs are good; doing monthly chemo
September	12	MRI results are good
October	21	8-month mark
November	14	MRI results show improvement from previous scan

2013

January	17	Planned trip to MD Anderson Cancer Center in Houston, TX, for a second opinion
February	6	Concerns begin regarding damage from chemo and radiation
	22	Second opinion in Houston; doctor recommends an unorthodox treatment regimen of Temodar with Accutane (acne drug); met with resistance by my doctor; we decided against this treatment
March	23	One year since diagnosis; feeling almost normal

July	11	MRI shows more improvement; another birthday; feeling good; give in to cake; start falling off Ketogenic Diet; eating sugars and starches again
September	12	Another good MRI; still feeling good; eating normally; not on ketogenic diet
November	14	MRI shows tiny spot; symptom-free, so not worried; enjoying holiday meals, but certainly not in celebratory mood
December	17	Additional growth but not in new area; change not dramatic but blood is drawn to resume chemo
	20	Symptoms flaring up again: limping, loss of grip in left hand, short-term memory loss, speech difficulty

2014

January	1	This year, we WILL find a doctor to remove tumor
	15	Caring bridge post invites friends to come see me; just lost friend to colorectal cancer; feeling low
February	11	Lab work not okay; low platelets and white blood cell count; deficits are occurring
	25	Tumor has grown and there's swelling; clear the calendar with plans for surgery
	27	Found surgeon who believed tumor was now safely operable using brain-mapping technique

March	5	Met Dr. Nader Sanai, Barrow Neurological Institute
	6	Plans in place for surgery; tests are done
	9	Rich's sister comes to town to take care of kids
	13	Tumor removed successfully
	14	Doing well; up and using a walker
	19	Discharged home from inpatient rehab
	31	Radiation and chemo starts; treating tumor bed and flair
April	17	Ketogenic Diet full-force now; also doing speech therapy, physical therapy
May	8	Hair loss started, decided to shave it all off; able to drive again
	15	Post-surgery MRI; CLEARED!
June	15	Vacation with the kids in Boston; left them with sister-in law; flew to Mexico for well-deserved couple's-only vacation
July	10	MRI shows everything is stable and unchanged

PART I

MY JOURNEY

CHAPTER 1

JUST A SMALL TOWN GIRL

My name is Melinda Ann Elwell, but everyone calls me Mindy or Min. I was born on a military base in New Jersey but our family soon moved to a civilian neighborhood in Massachusetts, near the Rhode Island border, when I was a toddler. My memories of childhood include all the fun of the 1970s: a split-level ranch house with a big playroom in the basement; orange shag carpet under every step I took; funky wallpaper on every wall; and lots and lots of packaged junk food and sugary powdered drinks I would never feed my own kids today.

We were a middle-class family and both of my parents worked hard to make sure their four kids had everything they needed for a modest, yet happy life. I have fond memories of summer vacations every July at a beach-house rental on Cape Cod and one vacation, in particular, when we saved all we could to visit Disney World at the cheapest time of year, August. As kids, we didn't care about the searing heat, the suffocating humidity, and not staying in the park itself. After a whole year of saving for this dream vacation, we were just glad to finally be there. The important lesson of patiently saving for a big reward stayed with me and is one I passed down to my own kids.

I met my husband Rich the month I started college at Bridgewater State University in Massachusetts. I was intimate with him from the minute I met him, but not for the reasons you might think. His fraternity pledge required him getting as many girls to sign their names on his bare bottom with a Sharpie pen. Mine was the first. I signed one of his still-barren cheeks, "Melinda," just to maintain some anonymity in case any of my dorm sisters would be the next one to have the Sharpie honor. I guess I liked what I saw because I sought him out soon after, and we began a relationship that has withstood not only Sharpies but also three C-sections and even terminal brain cancer.

Rich and I dated for a whole decade before finally getting married. I was busy with school, enrolled in a Ph.D. program right after graduating with a Bachelor of Science in Psychology and getting my Masters degree in Clinical Psychology. Marriage and our first son left me happy for my future. I had earned nine credits toward my Ph.D. but soon realized the importance of being a full-time mom. So, I left my job at a local detox hospital to give my first-born all the attention he deserved.

Rich and I soon bought our first house and were blessed with two more children. It wasn't until our third child was born when we decided to venture west and buy a house in Arizona. After some miserable New England winters that persisted through spring, and summers with too much humidity, rain, mosquitos and ticks, we decided our quality of life was somewhat compromised or limited on the East Coast. With three small children, we wanted to spend more time outdoors getting fresh air and exercise rather than being cooped up in the smelly, local YMCA while the snow piled up outside. We packed up our kids and the dog for a cross-country trek to start a new life in Arizona.

It was with plenty of tears that I said goodbye to my siblings and our parents, knowing how much distance would now lie between us. But I was excited to finally experience the other side of the country, lured by the promise of Arizona's climate and the beauty of our new neighborhood. It was a good move because, as it turned out, we were able to build our dream home a few years later, at the base of the beautiful White Tank Mountains, in the outskirts of Phoenix.

Our neighborhood is very unique and I believe the tranquility and peace of where we call home played a major role in my healing over the past two years. It has a small-town feel, modeled after a real town in Georgia, replicating the original style of the 1950s: we have a central square, numerous parks, a quaint fountain in the town common, perfectly green grass, tree-lined streets, a Main Street with shops, and a small health club and golf course. It's truly our little slice of heaven.

I shudder to think how much more difficult my recovery from cancer would have been if I had to be cooped up much of the year, as would have been the case if we stayed in Massachusetts. The mood of nature certainly affects my own mood. But, I suppose, if that were my reality, I would have learned to love even the East Coast weather somehow. Having terminal cancer made me appreciate everything that much more.

CHAPTER 2

THE GUESSING GAME

Five months before my forty-fifth birthday, the symptoms started. It was February 2012. Over the course of two to three weeks, I noticed strange sensations in my head whenever I turned around too quickly. If I could describe the feeling, it would be a sense of detachment, as though a part of my mind was lagging behind, trying to play catch-up with my body.

This alone wasn't enough to make me concerned, just curious. Then I started noticing the grip of my left hand become significantly weaker than my right. This was troubling because I'm left-handed. My writing started to become illegible, the letters I tried to form too small. As hard as I tried, I could neither control nor improve it. I did not know what to make of this. I thought, "Okay, maybe I need to switch up my grip and change the angle of my hand." I even wondered if it was merely the height of whatever table or counter I was trying to write on. I made adjustments but none of these changes helped.

A weakness on my left side, from head to toe, became noticeable next, but it was gradual, not all at once. I couldn't do my usual moves at the gym. This concerned me more and more, but not until two friends asked me why I was limping did I realize I should bring this list of weird and unexplained symptoms to a medical professional—but who?

4

I decided to reach out to Troy Anderson, my friend and former boss, who also happens to be a neurologist. After he read my email, he instructed me to make an appointment to see him as soon as possible. As I drove myself to Phoenix Neurology, I tossed around the possibility of living the rest of my life with multiple sclerosis. From what I knew of MS, the symptoms fit. I knew a few people who suffered from it. One particular friend is doing great; so well, you wouldn't even know she had MS if she didn't mention it. Another person I know with MS has an amazingly positive attitude, works full time and has tons of energy. Neither friend is in a wheelchair or struggling, at least not publicly. I decided I could deal with MS, if that were the case.

Troy initially mentioned MS as a possible diagnosis. After a neurological exam in his office, he admitted, "It could be a brain tumor, but I doubt it." Nevertheless, he ordered a STAT MRI, which our insurance company promptly denied. I spent the remainder of that Friday in my office, going back and forth between our insurance company and Troy's staff, begging for approval. By the time I achieved victory, it was too late to get on the schedule at nearby facilities. The soonest available scan would have to be scheduled at the only facility open on a Sunday—an hour away in the Valley. That meant two more days of waiting and wondering if I had MS or a brain tumor.

CHAPTER 3

THE FIRST AND WORST—MRI

The following Sunday, February 27th, Rich and our three kids drove an hour to Valley Radiology Center. When we arrived, there were no other patients in the waiting room and the receptionist was locking the door but, when she saw me, she quickly ushered me in. It seemed they were waiting for me, their last remaining appointment.

The kids and Rich proceeded to wait outside the building after I was asked to follow someone wearing green scrubs into a dimly-lit changing room which had lockers and a small sitting area. I'd been advised to not have any metal whatsoever on my body or clothes so I was dressed accordingly, in what would become my MRI uniform for future scans: a "lucky T-shirt," which was actually a sports bra, tank top, and yoga pants. I stuck my purse in the locker and plucked the key from its holding, dutifully following instructions as I knew there was no value in being overcome by fear.

The MRI tech asked me if I was claustrophobic. I didn't really know, having never been confined to such a contraption, so I didn't comprehend the importance of his question. I'm not sure what they would have offered me if I'd said, "Yes," aside from an anti-anxiety drug. Having now been through this experience, I highly recommend an anti-anxiety drug, or a less-restrictive, open MRI, if possible.

TIP: Take an anti-anxiety med for your first MRI, as a precautionary measure. You may as well be as relaxed as possible. If you fidget, it will interfere or compromise the accuracy of the scan, requiring a do-over. Get it right the first time, calmly.

I don't think anything could have prepared me for the frozen-in-time feeling of being in the MRI machine. Frozen, not in the sense of being cold, but rather paralyzed within its suffocating confines. The claustrophobic entrapment, mixed with the anxiety of what the scan would show, completely freaked me out. I still wonder if a little coaching beforehand would have eased my stress rather than going in cold turkey. But I suppose it may not have mattered, given the circumstances.

I jumped up on the table and positioned myself as instructed. After the technician made sure I was in the correct position, he started snapping things over my neck and head and attaching them to the table. He repeatedly asked me if I wanted music and, if so, what type. Apparently, this helps some people relax, not me, however. Music did nothing to minimize the craziness going on in my mind about being trapped like that. I had to come up with some kind of mind game, and fast. But I remember many intense waves of panic washing over me, crashing through every mental barricade I tried to put in its path. Being unable to see, move, or truly comprehend what was going on only added fuel to this panic. I'd never had such desperate feelings of helplessness before.

The technician spoke to me in between "pictures" and I could hear that he had a New York or a Boston accent. That gave me a little bit of nostalgic comfort but I still had moments when I felt I was going to lose it if I couldn't get up and escape from the imaging machine. I continued to dig into my mind and try to come up with a way to get through the process, which I was told would last about forty-five minutes to an hour. The tech instructed me not to yawn or swallow. Wouldn't you know it, if you are trying not to, the urge is irresistible. There were itches I couldn't scratch and coughs and sneezes I had to stifle. Oh, and that nagging urge to be done with it and get the hell out of there.

The first mental game that helped me keep it together was thinking about all of my friends and family. I named them in alphabetical order and simultaneously pictured their faces. I didn't want to miss anybody so I concentrated on doing a mental overview of the contact list on my phone, starting with "A" and acknowledging every person I could remember, all the way to "Z." One thing I realized was I had lots of friends named Amy, Tracey, and Jennifer. The call-up game worked. I think it was partly due to the reassurance of seeing their faces in my mind, reminding me how many special people I have in my life. I had so much time while the scan was completed that I repeated the process a few times. It was a good example of mind power, the power of intentional visualization.

When the scan was complete, the waves of panic immediately changed over to sweet relief. I couldn't get sprung from that vault fast enough. I remember naively thinking, "Thank God I'll never have to do *that* again." I didn't have any idea what to expect next but it quickly became clear I would not be dismissed as swiftly as I had hoped.

The technicians seemed hesitant, waiting for something, and they asked me for my neurologist's phone number. This triggered more anxiety. Two things were already wrong: I was having an MRI on a Sunday when most imaging centers were normally closed; and I was given a copy of the results on a disc to pass along to Troy, my neurologist, instead of being dismissed, empty-handed, to await the results in a few days.

Since it was Sunday, we all knew Troy wouldn't be in his office. But the technicians didn't know I had Troy's cell phone number and that I could reach him if need be. Since I had gotten the distinct message he needed to be reached immediately, I sent him some text messages and told him the imaging people needed to speak with him right away. My "Spidey sense" was tingling while I sat helplessly in the waiting room awaiting a reply from Troy. Eventually, Troy connected with the technicians and I was told to "run, don't walk" to his office first thing in the morning. Confused and concerned, I stumbled outside, now seeing the world in an entirely different light. Life would never be the same after this.

* * * * * * * * *

Rich and the kids had been waiting outside the MRI facility for a couple of hours by now. All they wanted to do was grab some takeout and go home. We drove to the nearest Panda Express in mixed silence. I can't remember how much was said along the way but I do remember a feeling of unusual quiet—as if a cloud of concern about what the technicians might have seen hovered in the car, the storm it promised too scary for discussion.

As we entered the restaurant (and I use that term loosely), a switch in my mind seemed to turn on. I can't explain it. Here we were, in a very basic, cafeteria-style establishment that looked just like any other Panda Express we had visited before, but this time was different. It seemed as if I was viewing my surroundings through a different lens. Something compelled me to take notice of everything in the place, including the decor on the walls and all the people in line. It wasn't that I suddenly became aware of restaurant design or now took interest in people watching; an inner command silently implored me to slow down. It whispered, "You may be in for a shorter life than you think. With your crazy pace, you're missing a lot of it."

This was just the beginning of my new, deeper vision, and the new appreciation for my surroundings, however mundane they may have seemed before cancer struck. At this point, I was still leaning toward MS as a probable diagnosis, swayed by Troy's shared suspicion. I started thinking about ways to cope with that. I knew, no matter what was afflicting me, I would fight it with a vengeance.

CHAPTER 4

DREADED DIAGNOSIS

The results of Sunday's MRI weren't available on Monday. The wait to uncover a diagnosis was now becoming torturous. I prayed I would hear something early Tuesday. The timing couldn't be worse because Rich was scheduled to go on a business trip to China that same day and he was wrestling with what to do. I urged him to keep his plans. No matter what we learned, there was really nothing we could do about it in the immediate future, and now it was even more imperative he not put his business in jeopardy.

He finally agreed and headed to the airport. I knew I'd be able to speak to him during his layover in San Francisco. If I didn't have any news by then, I'd have to wait another day for him to land in China to share it with him. It was an uneasy goodbye but I felt I could be strong.

I didn't have time to sit around and worry because Troy had ordered a series of blood tests. Just as I entered the restroom in the lobby of the lab, my cellphone rang. It was Troy. I had just spoken with him only a few moments ago. I wondered, "Why's he calling me now?" I remember his voice sounded strangely paternal. As I said before, Troy was my former supervisor and friend so I knew him quite well. This was odd. He wasn't curt but he took great care to say as little as possible over the phone, and ended the conversation shortly after it began. I realized two things: he has something really bad to tell me and I was really fortunate to have such a dedicated friend.

They couldn't draw my blood fast enough, because I knew Troy would be meeting me at home. As soon as they were done at the lab, I drove directly to my house, amazed at how my usual tendency to want to clean up the normal household disarray before a visitor arrived crossed my mind. I mentally slapped myself for such a petty and foolish thought in light of the seriousness of the situation. On the other hand, I tried to remain positive and somewhat normal. What a precarious balancing act that turned out to be.

My friend and neighbor, Sue, was one of the only people outside of my family I had told about my initial health concerns. She'd been in touch with me several times over the course of the morning to check for answers as I received them. Since Rich wouldn't be there to support me, Sue didn't want me to be alone when the MRI results came in.

Troy beat her to my house and started laying out the causes of my dizziness, balance issues, memory problems and the weakness on my left side. He was in the middle of his initial explanation when Sue finally appeared outside the sliding glass door. It was locked and that caused her to peer inside to get our attention. As I looked over, I saw dread quickly darken the expression on her normally bright, pretty face. I jumped up to let her in. After a quick hug, we made our way back to the couch and sat close, as if we were glued together. She immediately grabbed my hands and squeezed hard to brace us both as Troy continued, now ready to get to the heart of the matter.

As he resumed his explanation of what was going on in my head, all I could think about was my precious husband about to board a plane all the way to China. When would be an appropriate time to call him? Should I call him now and put him on speaker so he could hear the details too?

I forced my mind back to Troy's words, knowing I should just focus and listen. He started to describe different types and grades of brain tumors. *Did he say tumor?* My hand shot up involuntarily to cover my gaping mouth, but not before I inadvertently let out a shriek of disbelief. *Did he actually just say cancer?* I recognized the word "lymphoma" and knew it was associated with cancer.

Troy now started adding details to a diagram he started drawing, offering descriptions of the different grades. It all went over my head. I didn't want to hear details or statistics. I had the strongest urge to stop him mid-sentence and just ask, "What can we do about this thing? Tumors can be removed surgically, right?" Without hearing my silent question, Troy went on to explain the location of the tumor made it impossible to surgically remove without the possibility of paralysis. Then I heard him talk about the need to commence radiation and chemotherapy immediately. This was all was so foreign to me. I remember wondering how he could possibly be so sure what the course of treatment would be, based on one scan?

The next comment was even more disturbing. "This is treatable, not curable." All I thought was: "treatable," as in able to be treated; "curable," as in capable of being cured. The thought kept rewinding: *My brain tumor is treatable, not curable.*

As if this wasn't enough horrible news, he then informed me the size of the tumor was significant. I certainly wasn't expecting this. It was way more than I could handle at one time. I desperately needed Rich. I was quietly gasping for breath as I processed Troy's words, "We can't make this go away completely, but we can manage it for a time." On came the tears. I felt my body curl up into a fetal position. I started to sob uncontrollably, knowing I was in deep shit.

I looked over at Sue. She was crying and appeared to be in as much surprise as I was, shaking and speechless. All I knew was, I had to get Rich on the phone right away. His flight was boarding. I rose from the couch in a stupor and headed out to the back yard, phone in hand. Rich was about to board and answered. I couldn't waste time or mince words. I had to spit the news out of my mouth. I remember saying to him, "I've got the news. It's not MS." Immediately, Rich replied, "Well, what is it?" I blurted it out, "It's brain cancer."

I could hear Rich let out a cry and some other noises that were alien to me. I'd never heard him make such noises before, and I hoped I would never hear them again.

TIP: When you're about to get results of an important test, arrange for a stable and trusted friend or family member to be with you for moral support, to hold your hand, and to take notes. Don't try to go it alone.

---

* * * * * * * * *

The following is the initial finding from my first MRI, date of report March 8, 2012:

NEUROSURGICAL CONSULTATION: The patient is a 44-year-old left-hand dominant woman who is a patient of Dr. Patchell's referred for 1 month of progressive left hemiparesis, intermittent word-finding difficulty, found to have a mass on her MRI.

DIAGNOSTIC TESTS: MRI of her brain reveals right thalamic internal capsule enhancing lesion consistent with possible glioma versus lymphoma. Labs: White count is 7. Sodium 139.

ASSESSMENT: This is a 44-year-old left hand [sic] woman with left hemiparesis, leg greater than arm, intermittent word-finding difficulty with an enhancing right thalamic mass.

* * * * * * * * *

By the time Rich got back from China, we had a date scheduled for the biopsy: March 9, 2012. It was during this time that Troy and his wife came by the house for a visit. I was despondent about what the biopsy would confirm. As we talked, my fears about the kids' future were at the forefront of my mind and became the topic of conversation. The tears soon started.

Rich had to excuse himself for a quick drive to pick up our son from school. While the three of us were alone, Troy whipped out a piece of paper and started to draw a bell curve to point out survival rates. I'm sure he didn't realize how upsetting this visual was to me. He just wanted to point out the facts of surviving my type of cancer.

When Rich returned with Dom, my cries had escalated to a hysterical level that I could hardly control. Troy explained his bell curve to Rich. But I couldn't take any more information at that point. I felt my body shaking and rocking, my knees tight to my chest. I began to feel like a freak show and I wanted them to leave. I remember running to my bedroom, shrieking that I just wanted to be left alone for a while. The truth was, I already felt alone in a sense. I was now singled out with brain cancer, living in a nightmare and it was impossible to know what lay ahead for my family and me.

* * * * * * * * *

At the time, and for an entire year following this, I was blissfully unaware my prognosis was only eighteen months of survival. Although I knew the imminent danger of a malignant brain tumor, this time frame was never actually discussed with me directly. Rich knew immediately following my biopsy and assumed I was also told. We both avoided the subject for our own reasons. Looking back, it's still a mystery to me how this could have happened. I'm grateful it did, however. Had I known early on I was given only eighteen months to live, I would probably have reacted very differently to my treatments, and to life in general. I may have been inclined to give up. In my blissful ignorance of the odds, however, I fought. I believed it was possible I could win this fight.

The mind is a very powerful thing. While I understand doctors often give potential end points to patients with the best of intentions, I believe if it's at all possible to steer clear of defining someone's imminent death, it could possibly fuel a stronger will to overcome it. Not all will be as lucky as me, but it certainly helps boost the psyche of a patient.

Having been in this situation, I can tell you that, from a patient's perspective, there's enough bad news embedded within a malignant diagnosis of brain cancer. What harm would it do for medical professionals to refrain from defining a finite time horizon of survival? I know the statistics are out there. It's easy for anyone to look up survival rates and reach their own conclusions. But what if they don't want to? What if they don't want to know?

This may sound simplistic but, just as expectant parents may not want to know the sex of their baby until it's actually born, maybe it's best for a patient to just deal with one thing at a time—absorb the fact that you're in for the fight of your life, but that anything is possible with a positive attitude and a little encouragement.

The hope to overcome terminal cancer empowered me. Had I known the eighteen-month prognosis, I may have been resigned to ticking off the days instead—giving in to fear and giving up on life; what a shame that would have been, for me and my family. I'm living proof of hope. Eighteen months ended over a year ago and now, here you are, reading my book, and I'm enjoying life, my precious family, and every God-given day of my future.

CHAPTER 5

TELLING THE CHILDREN

At this point, we had every reason to believe our life, as a family would be drastically changed. Since my diagnosis would affect all of us, we knew the moment had arrived to share this horrible news, first with our three children. This was done without my involvement and without me being present. We decided it would be better that way. I was mentally and physically fragile, not speaking or hearing well, and still not prepared to discuss it, let alone help devise the best possible plan of outlining such news.

Given our children's ages at the time (13, 10 and 7), Rich didn't go into too much detail, except with our oldest son, Richie. Taking care to be sensitive to each child's level of emotional maturity, Rich spoke to each of our kids separately. With our oldest, he outlined all the facts surrounding the cancer diagnosis and prognosis. Rich remembers saying, "Mom has an aggressive disease and it could kill her." Then, he remembers crying and hugging Richie while he absorbed what he had been told.

TIP: Revealing difficult news such as a cancer diagnosis to children is a delicate matter. In our case, with three children of varying ages, we decided the healthy parent would be the messenger. The conversations were tailor-made to each child's understanding and given one-on-one, to allow each child their privacy.

With our other two children, Rich gave them just enough information that was appropriate for their age level. In preparation for writing this book, we asked each of the kids to write down their feelings from the moment they learned Mom had brain cancer. Their consensus answer was: very afraid, upset and confused. The thought of living in a world without their mother was terrifying to each. They had difficulty sleeping due to the ongoing stress about my condition. We also learned they carried this emotional burden with them every single day. Our youngest, Domenic, admitted he was reluctant to talk about it with anyone because he feared he would break out in tears at any moment.

The undercurrent of grief, especially for a child, is impossible to ignore. How they kept their fears and simmering emotions in check while they dealt with school, friends and their growing list of chores, makes me realize the resilience inherent in children. With an issue like cancer, we felt it was the right decision to be honest about the repercussions, albeit in a gentle fashion at first. It became a growth period for them as human beings and it also strengthened our family unit as a whole. Working together to get through that first year of my struggle made us bond in a way that transformed each of us for the better. We're certainly lucky for the outcome of my case but, had it turned out differently, at least our children would have had ample preparation for a negative turn of events. I sincerely believe putting everything on the table, from the beginning, prepared us all for whatever God had in store for our family.

I'd like to share with you the personal accounts from my husband and children, upon hearing the news of my brain cancer. This is one of the most difficult moments anyone will bear in life. These short essays were all written during the development of this book. Perhaps that's why Rich and the kids were each able to write so honestly. I'm sure if my health went according to the original prognosis, their answers would have been the same but they may not have been able to write them down. I'm grateful for this cathartic exercise because it allows me to see how each of my kids has matured, in line with my own physical strength after such a difficult journey in search of normalcy. If any of you, or your children and loved ones, are facing such a situation, you may relate.

From my husband:

When I heard the diagnosis, I was shocked and fell to the ground in tears. When the doctor spoke to me, he said, "We are going to beat this. Don't worry about it." But inside, I was terrified about what he had said.

The first thing that I was going to change was my schedule. I started working from home instead of at my office, about 15 minutes away. I went and talked to my employees about Mindy's diagnosis. I asked them to step it up as much as they could to help me out. I told them, "If you can't work some longer hours, then let's lock up the doors and we'll walk away," because I was willing to walk away to take care of Mindy. They did step up and helped me out, and we kept things going.

When I had to break the news to the kids, I spoke to each child at their level, according to their age. I told our oldest, Richie, everything. I told Angela, our middle child, what I thought she could handle but with less detail than our oldest. Domenic, at only nine years old, was told very little. We did not speak as a group. I talked to the kids individually.

I often felt overwhelmed and sad. I sometimes lost my faith. In trying to cope with all this, I drank more alcohol than was healthy. I just wanted to squash my emotions. In the morning, I would go to the gym with Mindy to find some balance in a normal routine and keep her spirits and our physical strength up as much as possible. I prayed a lot.

Every bit of good news became a milestone for us. My hope for Mindy was renewed each time she had a good MRI. We were also encouraged when we saw that we were growing from our challenges and pain. When Mindy became stronger and her hair grew back I felt better. I guess this made me feel I was seeing the light at the end of the tunnel.

There were some private moments between us when she wanted to discuss my life without her. We talked about the future of our family with just one parent. It was painful to think about but Mindy wasn't uncomfortable talking about it. I didn't like it at all. I was completely terrified about raising the kids alone and I didn't want to talk about it.

Looking back at what we've been through over the past two years, I realize there's nothing I would do differently if we had to go through this again. I think we handled it well. The biggest piece of advice I have for others: Be your own advocate. Ask questions. Do research and trust your instincts. Seek counseling if needed. There's no shame in that.

—Rich Elwell

From my oldest son, Richie, 17:

In my life there have been many difficult obstacles that I have had to overcome but the greatest of all obstacles was my mother's diagnosis. Two years ago I was told my mother was sick. I was told my mother has brain cancer. At the time I didn't even know what to think. I had no idea what cancer was like. All I knew was that it was a very serious sickness.

Before I knew what was even going on, both my mom and dad were going from doctor to doctor, professional to professional, to seek help while I tried to continue living a normal life as a high school student.

I learned about the diagnosis on a weekend and, on the following Monday, when I returned to school, I didn't know what to tell my friends or my teachers. What was I supposed to tell them? Should I just say to them, straight up, that I may not be acting normally because my mom was diagnosed with cancer?

I don't want anyone to feel sorry for me. I just want to be treated as a normal student. And, because of that, I didn't tell anyone. Even though I hadn't told anyone about what was going on in my life, I knew people would find out soon enough. One day, I couldn't turn in a homework assignment for my English class. I just told my teacher that I had family issues and I couldn't get it done in time. My teacher just thought I was being lazy and I just didn't do my homework because of that. I didn't try to reason with my teacher because I just didn't want to argue with anyone. But, after class, two people who knew that my mom was sick explained to my teacher that I really had a serious problem within my family and because of it I couldn't complete that assignment. And, because of this, many more people found out that my mom was sick.

Soon enough my mom's many friends came to our family's aid. One of my mom's close friends set up a system where people could sign up to deliver dinner for my family so we wouldn't have to worry, and it was my job to coordinate with the people delivering the food. There came a time when Mom was more capable of preparing meals so we put the meal delivery on hold. She seemed happy being in the kitchen again and helping make our dinners. She didn't want to seem like some sick person who can no longer do anything for themselves. She then asked the people to stop delivering us dinner. Although I liked to have dinner delivered to us every night, I can understand why she didn't want people to do this anymore.

Soon enough, my life slowly returned to the way it was before all of this happened. I returned to my school activities, doing homework, and after-school activities, and my mom returned to her normal activities as well. Even though I know that my mom is sick, I try to live with it and so far, that has worked out for me and I have been able to live my life without worrying too much.

I'm not uncomfortable talking about this. I admit I only prayed a few times because I never noticed a change due to it. Right now, I just appreciate my mom and dad. I know they are always here for me even though they are in their own battles. I try not to worry and be prepared to help a lot.

I feel like we are closer now because we spend a lot of our free time together. Plus, I'm older and I've matured since she was diagnosed.

— Richie Elwell

From my daughter, Angela, 14:

I remember feeling really sad when I heard the news of my mom's brain cancer. I understood the seriousness of the situation and I couldn't stand the thought of a world without my mom. I still can't, and I don't want to lose her.

That first night that I found out about it, I thought about what might happen if my mom wasn't there anymore. It was very hard to sleep.

I don't have any friends who have dealt with cancer in their families but I was scared by the stories on television. It always exaggerates some of the effects but it is still very serious. I talked to some of my close friends about it. I tried praying but I'm not really that religious. But I wanted to try anything I could, so I did.

When I was really upset about stuff going on I never did anything physically to lash out or anything. But I remember crying and being sad about it. I talked to my dad about it the most. He explained it to me and reassured me we would all get through this.

After going through all of it, I think it helped me be more caring for others because I had to help my mom with certain things. Right now, I'm not uncomfortable talking about it. It feels good talking about this.

One thing I learned about my parents, since all this happened, is how hard they work for us. They always do what's best for us and make sure we're okay and getting everything we need.

If I had to give advice to someone else my age going through something like this, I would tell them to stay strong throughout this process. It will get scary and sad at times but you just have to have faith.

Now that things are better, and we're getting through this, I feel that my parents are a lot more open and honest with me about everything.

—Angela Elwell

From my youngest, Domenic, 9:

When I first found out, I felt sad and scared that she would die, and I was really afraid. I didn't really know what it all meant because I didn't understand what was going on and I was confused. That first night, I was really worried and scared.

I didn't talk to my friends about it. Nobody I know had parents with cancer. I didn't want to talk about it anyway because I will probably have cried. I did talk to God about it and I was hoping that she would be okay and I worried a lot. I did talk to one friend about it the most.

When I was angry, I hit some pillows and sometimes I felt really stressed. It was weird having a bunch of other adults in my house cooking for us and washing our clothes.

At first, I was scared and sad but, as she got better, I felt excited that she was getting better and stronger. I was proud of her for fighting it so well.

I'm not really uncomfortable talking about it. A lot of people know about it already. It feels alright to write things down and I'm comfortable about it.

My dad went out of his way to help Mom and that makes me feel happy. We didn't have to help her like this before because we didn't have to.

If I had to tell another kid going through this something, I would tell them to help as much as you can, pause your video games and come home straight from school to help at the house.

Now that we're getting through this, I see my parents act the same now to each other as they did before. It doesn't really surprise me because I knew how they felt about each other before.

—Domenic Elwell

* * * * * * * * *

With regard to the rest of our family and friends, we decided there was no point in telling everyone we knew about the diagnosis. Rich made phone calls to my dad and to his own parents. My father, who lives on the East Coast, was shocked and tearful when he heard the news over the phone. My mom had breast cancer decades ago and, unfortunately, she succumbed to a serious depression and drank herself to death in 1994. The news of my cancer probably resurrected difficult memories for my dad.

Rich's parents were in disbelief and urged Rich to get a second opinion. The rest of our circle—friends and those in our church—were kept up to date through a "Caring Bridge" we set up online. On this website, we would share updates on my condition and treatments, visible to all who joined. Many people signed up to receive text alerts. The caring bridge became a convenient way to share good and bad news without the emotional charge of repeating everything, over and over, and hearing cries of shock or emotion.

When I regained enough of my speech function, I made my own phone calls, speaking with my siblings about the situation but sparing them some of the details. I limited my phone time to only those crucial calls because it was a real struggle to speak, both physically and emotionally.

One of the early realizations from my new state of arrested functionality was: I was much easier to find, usually in one of two places: in my bed, or on the family room couch. Being relatively immobilized allowed for more quality time with the kids, enjoying trivial entertainment that would normally not have been my cup of tea. After school, the kids were mindful to mark their list of chores off a dry-erase board, come find me on the couch or in my room, give me hugs, and share their school progress with me. They would stay nearby to get started on their homework and, on week nights, we would watch movies or television together. This allowed me to rest my mind and body yet still enjoy some lighthearted moments surrounded by Rich and the kids, without feeling lonely and depressed.

TIP: Set up a Caring Bridge online (caringbridge. org) so friends and family can be alerted simultaneously to news about your health. This will save you precious time on the phone and writing emails.

CHAPTER 6

NEEDLE BIOPSY

It was time to find out the specifics of my tumor. In order to get a sample for the pathology tests, a biopsy of the tumor had to be performed.

Before the biopsy could actually be done, the neurology team would need a second MRI, which was ordered immediately. These results confirmed a large tumor in a tricky location of my brain. The next step was to find out exactly what this mass was. On March 9, 2012, Dr. Kris Smith of the Barrow Neurological Institute in Phoenix, Arizona, drilled a small hole in the top and back of my skull. Because of its location, Dr. Smith had already determined there would be no attempt to actually remove the tumor. The risk of paralysis or the loss of other functions such as speech was simply too great.

This was certainly disappointing, to say the least. But, at the time, the diagnosis of brain cancer left me no choice but to follow the lead of the doctors and specialists on my case. This wasn't the time to be a renegade. After the cancer was confirmed, it took time for me to absorb it all. I trusted my medical team and followed their traditional treatment recommendations. But as much as I had confidence in the professionals, I remember feeling like a passive bystander in my own life.

I know I should have asked more questions about the biopsy procedure, but I was terrified about it. Having now been through it, though, I can say it was not as big a deal as my nerves made it out to be, although it required in-patient hospital care for a few lonely, delirious days. Also, there was really no getting around the biopsy; it was a necessary first step toward forming a strategy for my treatment plan.

Dr. Smith extracted a piece of the tumor with a thin sucking device inserted through a tiny hole he made, being careful not to interfere with any brain tissue and cause potential harm. He took enough tissue for two biopsies, one of which was submitted to Dana-Farber Cancer Institute in Boston, for a second opinion. The initial pathology from Barrow revealed Anaplastic Astrocytoma, Grade III (AA3). We got the corroborating results from Dana-Farber in Boston just days later.

I was still out cold from the anesthesia by the time Dr. Smith got the pathology results from the lab. It was at this point he told Rich I had approximately eighteen months to live. Rich remembers hearing, "Expect the best, plan for the worst." Not until I was finishing this book did I learn the specifics of that moment between Dr. Smith and my husband. Rich explained, "When I heard the diagnosis, I was shocked. When the doctor spoke to me, he said, 'We are going to beat this. Don't worry about it.' But inside, I was terrified." As it turned out, Rich assumed I was told the same thing so we never actually discussed it. I'm grateful for not learning of this for another year.

* * * * * * * * *

The following are Dr. Smith's surgical notes from the biopsy procedure:

Date of Procedure: *03/09/2012*

Preoperative Diagnosis: *Right enhancing thalamic lesion.*

Postoperative Diagnosis: *Right enhancing thalamic lesion. Frozen: Astrocytoma.*

Name of Procedure: *Right needle biopsy with wand guidance.*

Indications: *This is a 44-year-old female who had noticed slowly progressing hemiparesis on the left side. MRI showed that there was an enhancing lesion in the thalamus. The risks and benefits of surgery, including the risk of bleeding, infection, coma, paralysis, death, as well as biopsy not revealing the component were explained to the patient. She indicated she understood and wanted to proceed.*

Procedure: *The patient was marked in the preoperative area on the right side of her head where she was brought back to the operating room. She was intubated by Anesthesia. Her eyes were taped shut after ointment was placed. She was then transferred to the OR table where a Bear Hugger was placed on her lower body. Her head was then turned slightly to the left and her head was placed and secured into a Mayfield, with a bump under her right shoulder. The wand was then verified with a previous MRI that had been put into 3-D and it was verified in multiple points along her skull. We then found a good trajectory, and the patient was prepped and draped in the usual sterile fashion. We infiltrated the area was [sic] 1% lidocaine with 0.5% epinephrine.*

Then again using the wand we were able to identify a good trajectory. We used a vertex arm. We first drilled a small [sic] and then passed the vertex needle biopsy to the appropriate spot within the lesion. We took 2 biopsies, the first one and then the second one 180 degrees off the first one. They were both sent to Pathology, where the frozen came back astrocytoma. Once the frozen was back, we then replaced the needle and then pulled the entire biopsy needle out.

We then copiously irrigated the incision and removed the system. There was no bleeding. We then closed it with a single stitch of nylon, and the patient was removed from the Mayfield.

The patient was extubated without difficulty, transferred to the gurney and transferred of the [sic] PACU without problem. The attending was there for all critical portions of the case.

* * * * * * * * *

As I slowly woke up in the recovery room, I remember realizing what just occurred despite a very foggy mind and heaviness in my body. I threw up several times and tried desperately to focus my eyes. I vaguely remember seeing Rich, his best friend Steve, and Troy in the recovery room but they were very blurry. Nurses seemed to constantly hover around my bed, checking vitals and asking me to rate my pain level. I was soon wheeled into a private recovery room where I would spend the next few days.

Over time, I began to take notice of my body. Something strange was strapped to both my legs. It was initially very confusing. As I stared at these blue plastic wraps around my calves, I could feel them automatically squeeze and let go, continuously. I soon learned this was to maintain blood circulation and to prevent blood clots. That made a lot of sense given my immobility. It certainly wasn't unbearable—yet.

The next thing I realized was something in my nose for oxygen, and various needles, clips and monitors in different places, both in and on my body; and, of course, a catheter. Oh, how memories of having three C-sections came flooding back. As soon as I could string two words together, I asked when it could be removed. I wasn't thrilled with the answer: "Not today and maybe not for a few more days."

I was put on steroids right away to reduce swelling from the procedure. Common side effects from steroids include increased appetite and difficulty sleeping, perhaps even an increased sense of wellbeing. Not me, however. Maybe this was due to the fact that I was uneasy taking them. I knew the long-term use of steroids could be quite damaging. As it turned out, two weeks was the prescribed duration. I was grateful for that.

It was impossible for me to stand or walk on my own immediately following the procedure. Over the course of a couple of days, I got to my feet with the help of nurses and a walker, just so I could shuffle to the bathroom. We were hoping that standing would lead to walking. Soon, I started venturing through the hospital halls, aided by a physical therapist and Rich. A canvas-type, heavy belt—a "gait belt"—held me up while I gripped my walker. Talk about feeling helpless.

The staff took notice of our difficulties and encouraged me to join their inpatient rehabilitation program. No doubt the therapy rooms would be full of trained and capable professionals, along with the latest and greatest equipment. The only reason I declined was because I sorely wanted to go home. Physical therapy outside the confines of a hospital sounded more therapeutic and motivational for a true recovery. Before this could happen though, we needed to have a special meeting with a social worker and a nurse to prepare for my discharge and make plans for a physical therapy regimen.

* * * * * * * * *

Rich stayed overnight with me in the hospital those first two nights. After that, I insisted he go home. I couldn't stop thinking about the kids doing okay at home. They were only seven, ten and thirteen at the time. Old enough to know something very wrong was happening with Mom, but too young to realize how potentially tragic the situation really was. Rich agreed he should shift focus to the kids and left the hospital that third day.

All through our experience, Rich and I never neglected bringing our children into the reality of our family situation. Rich took the lead and, for that, I'm forever grateful. Looking back now, he's told me, "There's nothing I would do differently if we had to go through this again. I think we handled it well." Remembering those first few weeks, however, I wasn't sure what to expect about my kids' reactions and how they would handle any potential emotional scars.

The next day brought much-needed solace. Rich knew how badly I wanted to see the kids so, upon his return to the hospital that day, I was thrilled to see Richie, Angela and Domenic follow his lead right to my bed. To my relief, they weren't visibly upset, although I certainly wouldn't have blamed them. It's difficult for me to think about all the pain my children were dealing with at that time, facing the real possibility that terminal cancer may remove their mother from their lives. This visit in the hospital must have really driven home the seriousness of our new family situation. I'm sure, for them, it was a pivotal turning point.

In spite of my delirious state, I knew all too well the confusion that faced them. I was very proud of my kids. They seemed relatively calm and not too worked up about it. I learned later that Rich had explained the situation to each of them and gave them some forewarning as to what to expect, how I would look and so forth. Fortunately, by this time, the oxygen tubes were removed, but the blue leg squeezers were still attached. They had now become an irritating appendage. The automatic squeeze and release was beginning to wear on me, making me feel constrained and claustrophobic. I remember starting another mind game, this time to overcome the anxiety they were starting to cause. I would close my eyes and pretend it was just our little wiener dog, Tanner, cuddling up against my lower legs as he occasionally does when I nap on the couch. It was a small but sweet reminder of normalcy, a little bit of comfort in an otherwise shitty situation.

This discomfort was forgotten now as I was being rewarded with a beautiful moment the minute our three kids walked into the hospital room and hugged me. It was wonderful to see them acting normal, snagging food off my lunch tray, and asking lots of questions. I relished every second, although it was a brief visit. We reassured them I'd be home very soon. The physical therapist arrived not long after the kids got there, ready to march me down the hospital corridors and complete some paperwork. The shortness of the visit was for the best, however, because my tolerance for stimulation was very low, and Rich was irritable from lack of sleep. I could tell that stress was wearing him down. Even so, he rose to his usual level of composure and strength and shepherded all three kids out the door and back home to their new routine without Mom.

* * * * * * * * *

When the time finally came to review my discharge plan, our special meeting with those in charge went smoothly. Rich and I were confident in the benefits of being discharged directly home rather than to the inpatient rehab. The powers that be graciously agreed. They saw the emotional benefits from being surrounded by family and pets, and how that could be instrumental in my recovery. I can't tell you how thrilled I was when they started completing my discharge papers. However, it was contingent upon verification of insurance coverage for physical therapy at home. We found out this coverage was in place, thankfully, and my first appointment was scheduled. It was at this time we also reached out to a friend, Mitas Medrano, who was a physical therapist. Although she ran the Verrado Chirofit Chiropractic and Physical Therapy clinic just down the street from our house, she promised to come by each day after work for four weeks, at no charge, to help me get back on my feet. I was overwhelmed by her generosity.

One of the most difficult side effects from the biopsy was an almost-overwhelming fatigue. With Mitas' help and guidance, I was able to exercise almost every body part and somehow push through my urge to drop on the spot and rest. She sure wore me out, but soon I was doing knee bends, squat-type leg exercises, stretches and fine motor exercises for my fingers (squeezing and stretching squishy things). Mitas explained to me that we could repave weakened pathways in my brain with repetitive exercises that strengthened the left side of my body—my left foot in particular. This concentrated effort made a big difference in helping me regain confidence with a more balanced mobility.

While I began improving physically, I remember experiencing extreme sensitivity to noise and sudden movement. Whenever someone moved quickly around my field of vision, it made me uneasy. It took a while for this strange sensation to dissipate. Having three kids in the house made it difficult to stop sudden action all around me. Overall, I have to admit I actually didn't mind. For me, it was better to feel a little discomfort and relish my family's energy than to slip into a dark void of silence where my quiet mind could contemplate the loneliness of mortality. Being around my children reminded me I was fighting not just for myself but also for them.

CHAPTER 7

———

EASTER "VACATION"

Soon after this recovery period began, Easter loomed ahead, my first one as a person with disabilities. I'll never forget it, but at least now I can laugh about it. Rich's parents arrived for a two-week holiday visit. I normally would have welcomed their company but having an audience view my sadness and struggles, family or not, did nothing to help the recovery process or lift my spirits.

I know it wasn't their intent to be "voyeurs," but I couldn't help but feel like a one-woman freak show. It didn't take long for both Rich and I to feel the urge to scream, "You need to help us, not sit there and just watch! This is not the time for a vacation. Step up and do some dishes, clean something, or take one of the kids to the park." Of course, we didn't say any of these things. We kept quiet and stewed. In hindsight, we should have been direct and made our needs and wishes known with the understanding that they were in just as much shock about my situation as we were.

My advice to anyone dealing with a difficult physical recovery is to communicate in advance to anyone planning an extended stay, especially family. Let them know in advance this will be one time they will not be treated as "guests." Spare yourself from any weak links during your recovery. If an overnight visitor isn't capable of pulling their own weight, or is insensitive to your situation, recommend a short day-visit so they may show moral support, offer you a hug of compassion, get an in-person update on the patient, and then leave. Don't feel guilty about your personal space at this crucial moment in your recovery. The mental stress of an inconvenient visit when you're at your worst will diminish your recovery progress and sour your family relations.

* * * * * * * * *

One of the most painful and frustrating situations for me during this time was being dependent on the walker. Not only was it slow going, it was also awkward, frustrating and dangerous, especially with a more crowded house. The strain of using a walker found it's way into the muscles of my shoulders, neck and back, adding even more discomfort to my already–challenged body and psyche. I had no choice but to use it everywhere I went, whether at home or when venturing outside.

Since my in-laws were with us during this Easter holiday, we decided not to break the tradition of attending the Good Friday service at our church. Had they not been visiting, I suspect I would have forgone the service this year. We expected the crowd of Easter worshippers to be rather large, as usual, but we didn't anticipate how far away we would have to park from the entrance. I thought I could get along all right operating the walker from the car to the church but I was woefully wrong.

I felt like a public freak show, creeping along for all to see, and for all to pity; at least, that's how I felt in my incapacitated state. Some people hovered near me as I shuffled along, uttering a few kind words before they picked up their pace in order to find good seats before the service started. Others merely glanced my way silently and hurried past. Maybe they thought my condition was contagious. Truthfully, it was awful.

I could also feel Rich's tension. By the time the service was over, Rich and I were so frustrated by the whole scene and by the kids fighting that we were all practically in tears during the short ride home. It would have been better had we not have gone. Good Friday represented enough sadness without thoughts of my own death, triggered by the perceptions of those around me, seeing me in this condition for the first time.

On Easter Sunday, my sour mood persisted. The kids had gone through their baskets and now it was time to prepare our special Easter dinner. Being relatively incapacitated during such a special holiday, when my mom skills were usually in high gear, made me feel like a fifth wheel, utterly useless. In my attempt to be helpful in some way, I decided to tidy up the family room—with my walker. This was not a good idea. I wasn't used to sitting idly by while others tended to my house and my traditions. No matter my limitations, I felt compelled to at least be involved in the planning and preparation, even if they were minimal. This was one of those moments where the old me simply could not fathom the reality of the new me, what others called my "new normal."

As I shuffled about, determined to straighten up the disarray in one room, the front leg of the walker caught on an edge of carpet. Without my full mobility and muscle strength, I couldn't dislodge it. My frustration materialized into a spurt of energy, allowing me the strength to throw the walker, then myself, onto the floor. This was promptly followed by a rage filled sobbing session and, finally, a calm down and recovery. It was truly a tantrum but it taught us all a lesson, especially me. From this point on, I'd have to accept my limitations. I really had no choice. The only way I could find peace with this fact was to know and believe it would be temporary. I would make sure of that, somehow, someway.

By this time, we had already decided we would not be attending Sunday's Easter service. The events on Good Friday certainly cemented that decision. I just couldn't go through that again and neither could my family. Instead, we stayed home, had some friends join us, and Rich added his personal flair to our traditional side dishes, in preparation for our special dinner. It turned out to be quite the Easter feast— outstanding, and everyone had their fill.

You would think, by this time, it would have dawned on me not to feel guilty about letting others clear the table and do the dishes. I suppose years of being in charge of the kitchen were seared into my brain, even deeper than my tumor. After a couple of failed attempts to help, I was given a stern order to relax and let the guests fill in for me. As I look back on that time now, I wonder, "Why couldn't I just let others help? Why such a mental block about letting go? Most people would welcome the opportunity to take a pass from dish duty and sit on the couch." Soon enough, I got over it and found myself relaxing with my friend Chris over a glass of wine.

Later that evening, after our guests said their goodbyes, I tried a private trial run around my bedroom without the walker. While Rich was getting the kids settled for bed, I decided I'd try my luck at a couple of steps, unassisted. It was a small yet meaningful victory for my troubled mind as I stepped from bureau to bed. "Holy cow!" I thought. "It's Easter Sunday and I took a few steps!"

This gave me newfound hope, and an idea. I made plans to obtain a cane in hopes of discarding my dreadful walker. Our friend, Bernie, owned and operated a home-health staffing company for the elderly. Surely he would have a cane I could borrow. It would only be temporary, after all, I convinced myself. My plan was to use a cane until I gained more strength, balance, coordination and confidence. And that's exactly what happened. I admit, it was a little creepy when I received the cane and observed a sticker with a man's name and address on it. It was very likely the man whose cane I was clinging to was no longer among the living. Weird. Weird. Weird.

Moving forward with my goals, the cane was used in conjunction with daily physical therapy and trips to the gym. Soon, I stopped thinking of myself as someone on a downward journey toward life in a wheelchair. Progress was really happening. My goal of unassisted walking was becoming more possible with every passing day; what a major high point that would prove to be.

CHAPTER 8

BARROW NEUROLOGICAL INSTITUTE

Due to the results of the tumor biopsy, there was an urgency to begin radiation treatments, which would be in conjunction with oral chemotherapy. About a week before Easter, my treatments began. But there was plenty of planning to be done in advance of that. Having now known about my brain cancer for several weeks, Rich and I had lots of questions for the specialists. We wanted to explore every possibility for treatment, including diet, second opinions, surgery, etc.

The Barrow Neurological Institute (BNI) in Phoenix, Arizona, was the logical first step; it's world-renowned for cancer research and located close to our home. We were optimistic about potential options. Step one was getting in front of a neuro-oncologist.

Our first specialist was Dr. Roy Patchell, a well-respected neuro-oncologist and brain cancer expert. He had a reputation for reading brain MRIs with impeccable skill and had thirty-five years experience in the specialty of neuro-oncology. Unfortunately, Dr. Patchell wasn't open to discussing alternative treatments, supplements or nutrition. We assumed nutrition might not have been significantly emphasized in medical school curriculums at the time he was studying. That's probably changed now. But Rich and I did our research and believed the right diet and the right foods could make a big difference in optimizing my treatments, perhaps even diminishing some of my symptoms. We also wanted to learn about what foods should be avoided. It was worth a wholehearted attempt to learn as much as we could.

Solid answers to our basic questions that delved beyond traditional medical treatments were difficult to find, at first. It seemed conventional doctors were reluctant to "go there." We were surprised, given all the publicly available information we'd seen, such as how antioxidants (widely known to reduce cancer risk) should be limited during chemotherapy and radiation treatments. Could this be just the tip of the iceberg? We needed to chip away and dig deeper. We ended up finding two great resources at BNI, who answered all our questions about beneficial diets and adjuvant therapies: Leonora Renda, RDN, and Adrienne C. Scheck, Ph.D., whose valuable contributions you'll find in Part II of this book.

I would advise anyone who feels they're not getting enough answers to plow forward and persevere rather than become discouraged from investigating what lies beyond the scope of a particular doctor's expertise. As I found first hand, there's a wealth of information out there. You just have to be persistent and search for answers and methods that might alleviate symptoms, enhance your energy level, or even help minimize side effects. Relative to chemotherapy and radiation, I didn't think I had anything to lose by trying something new; in fact, I felt I had much more to gain, especially through the hope and spiritual well-being that accompanied knowing I was doing all I could to regain some semblance of a normal life.

During the discovery and treatment-planning phase that follows a definitive diagnosis, it's important to start interviewing other doctors so you have an alternative plan early on—before the time comes to make a change. Planning for second opinions from the beginning puts you on the offensive and minimizes hasty changes you might make due to emotional disappointments with your current medical team.

It takes time to build a patient-doctor relationship. The ideal doctor won't make you feel uncomfortable when faced with questions involving "gray areas." And it's important you not worry about offending anyone. After all, if you're in this position, it's likely your life is at stake. Don't be afraid to be your own advocate. You can certainly do so without being disrespectful. Increase your knowledge any way you can about treatment options, medical or nutritional.

Sometime after our first visit with Dr. Patchell, we learned he was no longer part of the practice and his patients were assigned to other doctors at the institute. My new doctor now became William Shapiro, a gentleman with decades of experience in neuro-oncology. At first, I was hesitant to ask him questions about alternative treatments, believing he would debunk them in favor of the traditional norms. After we got to know him, however, I realized he was open to discussing options, and this was comforting. There were times I actually jumped up and hugged him at the end of an appointment. It was also very humanizing to share some personal news beyond merely brain cancer, symptoms and side effects. I remember many pleasant conversations that ended with shared laughter. That makes a big difference to a family going through what we were going through. Over the next few months, we came to know each other and I felt supported and heard.

You, as a patient, should always be heard and feel like your opinions and concerns matter. The confidence you have in your medical team is one of the cornerstones of the healing process. Once you find a doctor you're comfortable with, one who will listen to you and answer your questions, it's important to be organized. Take notes and prepare questions for subsequent appointments so you can build on each session with additional knowledge.

There were many times I wanted to kick myself by the time I got home, realizing I hadn't made the most of my appointment with the doctor. I forgot to ask important questions or I was unclear about his answers and didn't record them for later clarification. The mental fatigue of worry, mixed with my physical weakness, put limits on my concentration. That's normal, but that's also why you should get in the habit of taking pen and paper to each appointment. We learned it's best to use one dedicated notebook, or a journal, to log information in chronological order. This makes it so much easier to chart your progress or check off your questions without forgetting something important.

* * * * * * * * *

Despite the privilege of receiving treatment at Barrow, Rich was curious to get a second opinion, for good measure. Through Rich's persistence, a sample of the tumor biopsy was also sent to the Dana-Farber Cancer Center in Boston. Being Bostonians originally, we knew of its esteemed reputation. Dana-Farber's results mirrored those from Barrow's team: there were no errors with the typing of the tumor, it was indeed an Anaplastic Astrocytoma, Grade III. While this isn't the most aggressive type of brain tumor, it certainly is malignant and deadly.

Regarding second opinions and insurance coverage, be sure to call your provider and make sure they'll cover the cost of the second opinion. It's a real possibility they may not. In any case, if you are covered, you'll probably need approval before additional tests can actually be done. Protocol, according to the insurance company's terms, is important. My tumor was discovered before Obamacare and, thankfully, the second opinion was covered. I believe it's expected, particularly with such a serious diagnosis that may require expensive chemo, radiation, and even surgery.

Speaking of surgery, be sure to confirm both the hospital and the neurosurgeon are "in-network" providers. If they're not, you'll wind up with a huge bill. In any case, co-pays can be ridiculously high as well, depending on your coverage, from prescriptions to MRIs and office visits. Check this out thoroughly ahead of time for some peace of mind and budget planning. Luckily, we ended up with a better plan with Obamacare, one that covered all the post-surgical therapies I was prescribed.

* * * * * * * * * *

The following is a Neuropathology Report of the frozen section taken by Dr. Kris Smith in the needle biopsy performed March 9, 2012:

Specimen Source:
1. Right thalamic enhancement, FS
2. Right thalamic enhancement

Clinical Diagnosis:
Brain Tumor

Gross Description:
1. Received fresh for intraoperative evaluation and labeled with the patient's name and "right thalamic enhancement" is a 1 x 0.2 x 0.1 cm portion of tan-white soft tissue. Smear slide is prepared. The specimen is entirely frozen on one chuck.

FROZEN SECTION DIAGNOSIS:
INFILTRATING GLIOMA, FAVOR HIGH-GRADE.

The previously frozen section is subsequently submitted for permanent.

2. Received in formalin and labeled with the patient's name and "right thalamic enhancement" is a single portion of tan-pink focally hemorrhagic soft tissue measuring 1 x 0.2 x 0.1 entirely submitted in cassette 2A.

MICROSCOPIC DESCRIPTION:

1, 2. Microscopic examination reveals a moderately cellular tumor most consistent with infiltrating glioma. The tumor cells demonstrate hyperchromatic oval nuclei with moderate atypia. They are embedded in a fibrillary background. Scattered mitotic figures are seen at up to 3 mitoses per 10 high power fields on the frozen section material. Neither microvascular proliferation nor necrosis are identified. A final diagnosis will be issued pending special stains, including a MIB-1 labeling index.

DIAGNOSIS:
(PROVISIONAL)

1, 2., RIGHT THALAMIC ENHANCEMENT, BIOPSIES:
INFILTRATING GLIOMA, FAVOR ANAPLASTIC ASTROCYTOMA, PENDING SPECIAL STAINS AND MIB-1 LABELLING INDEX.

The following is the Addendum Neuropathology Report, dated March 15, 2012:

ADDENDUM DISCUSSION:
A GFAP immunostain is performed on parts 1 and 2. The tumor cells demonstrate strong immunoreactivity for GFAP. The calculated MIB-1 labeling index is 8.9%. Overall, the histologic features are most consistent with an anaplastic astrocytoma.

ADDENDUM DIAGNOSIS:
1, 2. RIGHT THALAMIC ENHANCEMENT, BIOPSIES:
INFILTRATING GLIOMA CONSISTENT WITH ANAPLASTIC ASTROCYTOMA (WHO GRADE III).
- MIB-1 LABELING INDEX = 8.9%.

CHAPTER 9

PAPERWORK, SCHMAPERWORK

Before any of my treatments would begin in earnest, there were plenty of phone calls to the insurance company and paperwork to be filled out. In fact, it was standard procedure to fill out new paperwork prior to almost every appointment with doctors and specialists. It just seemed to be a huge waste of paper and time, although I understand a lot of it is required for compliance with privacy laws, malpractice insurance, record keeping, and diagnostics. But, nevertheless, it becomes a cumbersome drag for a patient to do this every single time. In my case, we were talking months into the future, if not years. I could imagine a mountain of paperwork would be built in that time span, and there I would be, a puny patient engulfed in the arms of HIPPA, not able to see the forest through the trees.

The good news is, once I became familiar with my new routine and with the very hectic pace of the medical professionals around me, I started to empathize even more with their rules and procedures. These dedicated, hardworking pros are truly spread thin. I have the utmost respect for them. My advice to anyone at the beginning of this routine is please be patient and go with the flow as far as following your institution's procedures. They are merely complying with the law and the staff is very likely in your corner, there to help save your life and ease whatever fear or discomfort you may have. With that in mind, if your initial reaction is like mine, it's normal and it will likely pass.

I would soon become a frequent visitor to the neuro-oncologist's office. He became the "captain of the cancer ship," in my eyes, the guy in charge. When I was a newbie, I carefully filled out every form the receptionist welcomed me with. I honestly believed somebody read and reviewed them prior to my face-to-face with the doctor or nurse so they could incorporate them into my treatments or discuss my concerns. It was disappointing to realize, however, this wasn't always the case. I doubt anyone really read my answers, at least in the beginning. I'm sure they face a pile of paperwork for each of the many patients they see every day but, in this case, the questions and answers were specific to a current condition or concern on the part of the patient and his or her treatment. Why bother with the paperwork at all? Why not just go down a checklist with each patient, one-on-one, so issues can be addressed as they come up during each visit?

The rising tide of paperwork and the constant flow of patients makes it more likely patient concerns could be overlooked, at least during your visit (this information is usually entered into your computer file later so the doctor has a record of everything). Early into my regular visits, I realized the answers I gave to their "clipboard questions" weren't immediately reviewed by the staff. I remember sitting down and checking off all the symptoms I had experienced over the past seven days, including unexplained itchiness, dizziness and headaches. When I saw the doctor and he didn't bring them up, I thought this meant they were of no concern. But a week or two after the appointment, a letter from the clinic arrived in the mail, recounting a summary of my last visit: it reiterated the "patient reported no problems." I pictured the computer data entry person buried under a white pile of pulp, gasping for air.

That's when I realized to never take it for granted the answers on these forms have been seen during your visit. It's best to verbally address every concern you have directly to whomever treats you that day. Rich and I tried a little experiment on a subsequent visit. Having settled down with my clipboard of forms, I signed every single one of them "Mickey Mouse." Sure enough, no one got the joke because no one noticed. Rich and I got a laugh out of it though, one of the first hearty laughs I'd had in a while.

As grateful as I am for the medical care of these good people, I do believe there are many inefficiencies and oversights in the healthcare protocol—that's just the nature of the beast. It's a well-meaning system, with communication channels and detailed forms listing every possible question or concern a patient may have. But my conclusion is it will always remain the duty of the patient to make sure the doctor doesn't miss something very serious.

We must each be our own advocate. Never shy away from speaking up about your symptoms. The medical profession, and cancer professionals in particular, face an almost overwhelming amount of patients every day. With the intent to see everyone that comes through their door, sometimes details you write down are overlooked. What I've found though is they will always listen and address what you tell them face-to-face. So never let that moment go to waste.

CHAPTER 10

YOUTH IN ASIA? NOW I GET IT

The most important paperwork of all were those grown-up documents most couples procrastinate on completing: the declarations that speak for us if, God forbid, something happens to us and we can't speak for ourselves. A will or a "Do Not Resuscitate" order (DNR) don't often rise to the top of our priority list when we're healthy and in our prime. In many cases, these important papers aren't considered and filed until we have children, which gives plenty of motivation to take care of such vital issues. I admit, Rich and I kept putting this off. Who really wants to think about death and dying? Occasionally, the topic would be kicked around among our friends but it seemed the majority of them only talked about it and, like us, kept putting it off.

It wasn't until just prior to my second surgery, the craniotomy, that Rich and I finally completed all the paperwork for a medical power of attorney for both of us. I was quite firm about what I did and did not want to be done in the way of heroic life-saving measures. It was a major relief to have it signed, delivered and filed. I won't deny, it was also very sad.

Brain cancer invokes a horrible fear. Being faced with the real possibility of decline and early death, I decided I would retain control of anything I could, even if I couldn't speak. A feeding tube would not be in my future. The last thing I wanted was to be a burden on my family. If my tumor would become unstoppable, the pain of watching my slow and painful demise would be enough torture for my husband and three children. No. This was not an option. I'd make sure of that.

In my former career, working as director of social services at a nursing home, I became very familiar with the information required to make informed, end-of-life decisions—namely, Do Not Resuscitate orders. Many DNR's were filled out on my watch and I was responsible for explaining all the implications to the families of our patients; what a huge responsibility that was, guiding the next-of-kin through this process. Now, faced with my own end-of-life decisions, I knew exactly what I needed to do. I drew on that knowledge and experience, although it didn't make it any easier.

* * * * * * * * *

I had a flashback from years ago and remembered the first time I heard the word "euthenasia." It happened when I was attending Bishop Feehan High School, a Catholic school. Naturally, religious education classes were required. Teenage students got their dose on Sundays. On one such day, my attention wandered during the lecture. As I tuned back in, I thought we somehow digressed to youth in Asia. I was curious to know why so I snapped to pretty quickly thinking, "Now, why in the world are we learning about the younger set in Asia?" I thought about it silently, trying to catch up to the class. I caught on eventually but, at that age, I remember the depth of the concept went completely over my head.

During future lessons, we also studied Elizabeth Kubler-Ross and the five stages of grief she discussed in her book, *On Death and Dying*. Her theory seemed logical, as I got further along in my reading.

A light bulb went on. Euthanasia, Dr. Death, or Dr. Kevorkian would put someone out of his or her misery, just as one might euthanize a sick or fatally injured animal so they wouldn't suffer. It seemed rather humane and compassionate.

Being a young and naive high-school student, I couldn't yet draw parallels to a human life, let alone my own life, nor could I understand why this topic would be relevant to a teenage girl. The only death I had experienced up to that point was the loss of my great-aunt Helen when I was in eighth grade. Aside from that, we lost our sixteen-year-old dog, Habu. Auntie Helen died of old age but Habu had to be put down.

Years later, while I was in my mid-twenties and working at the nursing home, death and dying surrounded me on a daily basis. I witnessed many deaths as a result of a variety of causes, including old age, of course. This led to my belief that whatever could be done to provide reasonable care and comfort for a dying patient should be done. It seemed more humane to me than prolonging their suffering through extreme efforts, many of which I witnessed in my profession. For the most part, trying everything and anything to keep death at bay seemed heartbreaking for the families and, more often than not, the patients were too far gone to be conscious of these attempts. It seemed they had already crossed the line of no return.

Seeing my own "point of no return" possibly looming in the horizon brought these memories to the forefront of my mind. If my time comes sooner rather than later, the DNR we put in place would ensure a natural passing—one divined by God. We, as a family, fell back on our faith that He would take care of me, and my destiny, not machines.

Along that same line of thinking (even though I will admit to a fleeting thought of suicide during the earliest, darkest days of fear following my diagnosis), this was ultimately not an option for me. One reason was deeply rooted in my belief in God. The other four reasons are the faces of my three children and my husband. It's heartbreaking enough for them to know my life is at risk from an unseen killer. It's quite another for me to abandon all hope of a miracle that there might be a doctor or a procedure we haven't yet discovered that could possibly remove, reverse or suspend the tumor's growth and allow me to outlive the early prognosis. That's ultimately what happened because we, as a family, hung in there and kept searching for hope. I desperately wanted to see my kids grow up. I desperately wanted to be brave rather than give in and impose death on myself.

* * * * * * * * * *

This is not a subject on which I, or anyone, can preach to another. It's a deeply personal issue. In speaking for myself, I'm not judging others. Not all cancer patients have family support. Not all cancer patients see a glimmer of hope, or believe in God and miracles. For some, the disease has already brought them to the point of no return with a stage of cancer that's completely untreatable. In this case, it may seem humane—for themselves and for their family—to initiate their own death, before the height of the natural degeneration and excruciating suffering begins.

Being diagnosed with Grade III Anaplastic Astrocytoma, I totally understand this. The chances of death are real. However, if I had gone down that road of premature self-destruction, I would never have found Dr. Nader Sanai, who successfully removed my initially inoperable tumor. Hearing his optimism certainly offered me hope and promise, a return to a quality of life I could live with.

The reality of my situation is that even with the tumor removed, the chance of rogue cancer cells rising up to pose another threat to my body still lingers. To combat that risk, I'm following a diet that's been proven to help brain cancer patients. I don't have many other options left. I've already had a lifetime's worth of radiation treatments. While chemotherapy is still an option for me, in the instance it's warranted (and it currently is), the diet seems to be working. I've had two MRIs since my tumor resection surgery in February 2014 that showed stability—great news.

I'm confident the life God has given me is being lived to the best of my ability. I cherish every month and year that goes by. The peace I have is difficult to explain in words. The bottom line for me is seeing the pride with which my children and husband look at me. The great appreciation we have for our time together, and the bravery I've shown them by fighting this thing called cancer, has brought us closer than any of us could have imagined. Whatever happens now is God's will, one we're ready to accept. I can truly say I can live with that and so can they.

CHAPTER 11

"BEAM ME UP, SCOTTY"

Now that the treatment plan was complete and the insurance coverage was in place, preparations were being made for an intensive round of radiation: a seven-week cycle that would encompass thirty-three sessions, five days a week, with oral chemotherapy taken daily during that time.

The first order of business was getting fitted for my radiation mask. This mask was created while I lay on a metal bed and technicians molded the material around my face and head. There were holes in the mask through which they would point the radiation beams toward the tumor and surrounding tissue. The set-up was a claustrophobic experience because I was strapped onto the table for what felt like a very long time and my eyes were covered while the mask was being molded. So, there I was, stuck, and not able to see anything, but I could hear their voices for a while until they would all suddenly disappear and leave me there to wonder what was going on.

I recommend learning about the mask-fitting procedure before actually going through with it. Had I done that, it would have reduced my anxiety. After the mask was completed, an MRI was performed to enable proper mapping of the beams. Overall, this was a lengthier process than I had expected but, as you can imagine, it was one of crucial importance.

TIP: Ask for a run-down of the radiation mask fitting procedure before you do it. It's tedious, you'll be strapped in place, and your eyes will be covered. This will be followed by a test MRI. An anti-anxiety med an hour before may help you relax.

---

* * * * * * * * *

Rich and I would make the voyage to the radiation clinic five days a week for almost seven weeks. Although the clinic was only a half-hour from our home, we allowed extra time to reduce any potential stress. In order to make sure we could achieve this, we had to schedule my daily appointment time. It was very helpful to be informed we could ask for the same time slot each day so we could get into a routine and minimize the impact on our family life. With three kids to send off to school, we wanted to avoid the morning commuter traffic. It felt like a small victory being approved for a treatment time of eleven in the morning. Having some control and a regular routine was important for us, especially during this early stage of treatment.

A typical radiation day would begin with a ring or a nod. In other words, when we entered the clinic, I would ring the bell if no one was in sight or, if there were someone behind the glass, we would secure a visual check-in. This acknowledgement was necessary because, otherwise, it was a crapshoot who would be called, and in what order.

It was like clockwork, for the most part. We usually got in and out with enough time for an errand or lunch.

A couple of times a week, we would have enough time to stop at Rich's office on the way home so he could check in on things and have a quick meeting with his staff. The impact of my treatments on the business was minimized because of the strong support from his employees. When I was first diagnosed, Rich announced the news to everyone at the office right away. His work schedule was the first thing to change. He remembers asking his employees if they would be able to step up their responsibilities while he cared for me. He admitted right then that, if this wasn't possible, he was prepared to lock the doors and walk away from the business in order to take care of me. This undeniable support from my husband never ceases to amaze me. Of course, all his employees were eager to work longer hours and do whatever they could to take the pressure off of Rich. With their support, the business continues to be strong and there were minimum interruptions over the past two years since my initial diagnosis.

It helped that the office was only fifteen minutes from our home. During our visits after radiation, I was able to stretch out on the couch in the front office while he tended to his business matters. The unfailing Arizona sun would warm me through the huge windows and help lull me to sleep very quickly. It didn't take long for me to realize I should listen to my body. I stopped fighting the urge to nap, even if that nap would be at the office. As a result of going with the flow of things and resting without worry, I was in a better frame of mind and felt rejuvenated throughout the day.

Our routine became so *routine* that, on most days, we could do the radiation, errands, lunch and business, and still get back home in time to relax a bit before the kids had to be picked up from school. While it's true that we fell into this routine only because we had no choice, it still amazes me how quickly we can adapt to even the most volatile changes in our lives. When it's a matter of life and death, the will to overcome any obstacle soon takes precedence over the inconvenience of the obstacle itself. Even so, I know we may be luckier than some; without the flexibility of Rich having his own business, this would have been much more difficult.

As if understanding the potential stress of disrupting our lives, several friends offered to step in to accompany me to the radiation clinic. This was a sweet gesture that I'll never forget. The family soon stepped up as well. When my father came to visit, and when my in-laws were in town, they each took Rich's place for a couple of treatments so he could have some full days at the office. These little moments of normalcy were healthy for his mental wellbeing.

It was at this time that I began to notice our family members, especially our parents, seemed to feel particularly scared and helpless. It was evident their anxieties were calmed when they accompanied me to the clinic. I suppose this symbolized a concrete contribution toward my recovery. Their willingness to participate so boosted my spirits, I treasured this time alone with them and I hope I made that clear to them at the time.

* * * * * * * * *

One inexplicable event occurred after my first radiation treatment. I had just finished my session, which was followed up by lab work, an appointment with the radiation oncologist and an appointment with the neuro-oncologist. This made for a very long and exhausting day. It was made even more stressful because, although I didn't feel any sensation during the treatment, I could smell this funky metallic odor and hear lots of buzzing and clanging while the table I was laying on rotated a couple of times. The radiation techs talked to me and this helped the time go by.

On this first day of treatments, I was also feeling a bit overwhelmed by it all. During the appointments, we had many questions for the doctors, most of them leading to even more questions and confusion. As I sat there, quietly listening to the dialogue between the medical professionals and my husband, I remember shifting my gaze to the floor and imagining myself slowly fading out of my own life. It was a surreal moment. I was stricken with the knowledge that there was a thief in my brain, robbing me of everything I held dear. If we weren't successful, this thief would eventually take over and gradually cast me out. Knowing I'd have seven weeks of this routine suddenly made it a daunting reality. Not having a guarantee that it would work made my mortality even more difficult to ignore.

By the time we were done at the clinic and the hospital, Rich and I were both feeling tense, hungry and scared. Our focus zeroed in on getting home to our kids and having dinner. We were mostly silent as we made our way to the tiny used car we purchased a couple of months ago. As we merged onto the highway, the car suddenly stopped. There was no noise or any indication of a problem. It just stopped. To make matters worse, the location where the car stopped was anything but ideal. Big, scary trucks and harried commuters in cars were speeding past us during rush hour, coming perilously close to our disabled vehicle. We were stuck around the corner from a sharp curve of an on-ramp. The sun was setting right in drivers' eyes and this probably made us even more difficult to spot. I remember thinking we would have felt much safer in our big Suburban. Our used Kia Rio was great on gas but uncomfortably tiny. And it chose the worst possible place to break down.

After attempting to restart the car a few times, unsuccessfully, Rich got out to look under the hood. The speeding trucks whizzing by shook our stranded "Hot Rod" (our nickname for our lil' car) and I remember sitting there realizing with dread that the glaring sun was making it almost impossible for oncoming vehicles to see us there. I prayed, "Oh, my Lord, please don't let that happen! My precious husband won't have a chance!" I felt my heart rate quicken and a sense of panic set in as I realized what could happen if hit from behind. Being partially under the hood, Rich could be run over.

All I could do was sit there, pray, and watch. For all intents and purposes, I was paralyzed. My motor functions were debilitated by the tumor and the walker I required for mobility was in the trunk. The realization that we could both be killed in an instant stung so sharp and deep, the irony was too much to bear. I started thinking of our kids and our already-tragic situation. I kept praying furiously, unrelentingly. Then, for no logical reason whatsoever, the engine turned over.

This was nothing short of a miracle. "What just happened?" we both were thinking. How and why did the engine start when all the previous attempts did absolutely nothing? It was utterly inexplicable. Rich and I were able to finally take a deep breath and regain a sense of calm. Not for long though because the car died again, not too far down the road. This time, however, we were able to call the highway department since we weren't in a perilous spot like we were just moments before. After twenty minutes, an officer arrived and offered to push our hot rod to the next exit with his car. It was a strange feeling being pushed like that but, nevertheless, it was a huge relief just to be safe.

I made a couple of phone calls: one to my dad, who was in town for a visit from Rhode Island and watching the kids; and the other to my friend Stacy, who kindly agreed to come and get us. We left the Kia at a repair shop near where the officer pushed our car. Exhausted and dehydrated, we finally made it home.

This was certainly not the outcome I had imagined for my first day of radiation. By now, we were beyond frazzled. But I couldn't help but see, through all the harried events of the day, the symbolism behind the small miracle we'd just experienced. Among all the other feelings I had that day, this roller coaster ride at the end was really an enormous sign of promise. I was compelled to pick up an inspirational book and relish in this amazing karma. Once situated comfortably, I was finally able to calm down and really think it through. The palpable memory of our close call and ultimate "rescue" warmed my soul. It gave me hope and reminded me to pray. Rich and I were momentarily immobilized, facing death right in the eye. I prayed because it was all I could do. That's the moment He rescued us. He answered my prayer. It's as if God was reminding me, just at the right time—at the beginning of my cancer journey—that anything was possible if I continued to have faith. So I did. And I still do.

* * * * * * * * *

A seven-week commitment isn't always easy to adhere to, even when it's something fun and exciting. It's a big chunk of time, especially for two adults with a business and three kids. But Rich and I had no choice with regard to the radiation treatment schedule, so we tried to make it as enjoyable as possible and take advantage of comic relief whenever it presented itself. I can't stress enough how important it is to have someone around you during this difficult time, someone who is positive and makes the best of things. I still needed to laugh, even though I had a brain tumor. And Rich benefitted from a good laugh too. We never lost our sense of humor. Actually, a little laugh is like a big dose of medicine.

The routine itself was really not that uncomfortable, and it quickly became familiar, except for my new role as an incapacitated passenger rather than my customary spot of being in charge and behind the wheel. During our normal, pre-cancer routine, Rich would often need to make business calls or check emails, which he could do while I did the driving. After cancer, that luxury became a thing of the past. This was a detour that was unavoidable and everything else took a back seat, so to speak. Things would get done, but within their new order of priority.

I didn't like contemplating the possibility of never being able to drive again. During our daily commute, however, my mind would invariably wander toward all the new "what if's" that accompanied a cancer diagnosis. Thankfully, my natural inclination to always see the glass as half full enabled me to ultimately shake these depressing thoughts out of my head. It also helped that we had a short ride to treatments, which gave me less time to have such sad thoughts. By the time we would arrive at the clinic, I'd usually find my healing mindset, just in time to absorb as much beneficial energy as I could from the radiation beams coming my way, so I could channel them toward that tumor I was going to destroy.

* * * * * * * * *

St Joseph's is an older hospital; how old, specifically, I don't know, but I could tell by the floors, the walls, and the bathrooms. To remedy this, parts of the hospital were being re-done or updated. I remember hoping the clinic was next in line for a makeover. It's a popular place, likely because of the great level of care they administer, as well as the population boom in the Phoenix area.

The radiation clinic itself was a small, one-level structure with an even-smaller parking lot. On any given day, it seemed hundreds of patients paraded through the door to enter "the vault." I thought it strange that the parking lot was so small but we quickly realized that, with patients rotating through every twenty minutes, the parking spaces freed up rather quickly. I remember thinking, "How odd for Rich and I to be discussing such mundane things as parking spots." But this hopping place was sure crowded. On the days when we visited the lab for simple blood draws and doctor visits, we'd park in the garage or splurge on the convenient valet service; at only four dollars, it was an economical treat.

Despite our determination to stay positive, Rich and I were seeing glimpses of cancer being a big business, and we started talking about that realization. Staying positive is one thing; being realistic is quite another. As sweet and friendly as they were at the front desk, we couldn't help but sense their very routine nature. Let's face it, they're employees of the business of cancer. There's nothing wrong with that. We certainly appreciated the fact that they were there to help us deal with our business of destroying cancer. It was just an interesting observation on our part that they had become almost casual bystanders amidst hundreds of patients who all have a potentially deadly disease. It's natural to become desensitized to what we see everyday. It happens to all of us, even me, as I realized that night in the Panda Express when it seemed like I was seeing it for the first time in my life. It took a cancer diagnosis to snap me out of my desensitized mode. If taking it in stride was the modus operandi that worked for some in the clinic, perhaps it was like a protective persona that shielded them from the harsh reality of their occupation. I can't say I blame them. I began wondering if the techs ever ran into former patients out in public. I also thought about the visible decline of patients and whether or not the techs thought to themselves, "I've seen this over and over, and I know what's coming. Today, it's a cane, next week, it'll be a wheel chair…"

The most important things of all, however, were the attitudes and skills of the radiation oncologist and those of the scientists designing my mask. Of course, I expected a team of highly intelligent, engineering, science-types planning and mapping out my treatment mask. Putting our trust in these nameless, faceless people whom we would likely never meet, I would soon be adorned with my radiation mask—the fruits of their expertise, to be beamed thirty-three times in total.

* * * * * * * * *

We called it "the vault" for a good reason. The four-inch thick door led (no pun intended) to the radiation room, through which I would soon be escorted. With my mask in place and my body snapped onto the table, the techs would then flee from the room to administer the treatment from the "safe" side of the massive, heavy door. Now, I'm a smart girl, but I couldn't figure out how it was therapeutic (or safe) to receive massive doses of radiation and come out seven weeks later no worse for wear. At this point, I had to simply believe what I was being told—that radiation shrinks the tumor while the chemo does its thing simultaneously. I understand the scientific evidence of this treatment but, for a patient going through this, it's still difficult to not wonder if healthy tissue is being harmed in the process, possibly beyond repair. I would soon find out. Now I know first hand why one of the scariest parts of cancer is the traditional method of treating it. I've heard many say, "If the cancer doesn't kill you, the chemo just might." Well, radiation is pretty harsh too, more on that later.

All these fears aside, I began to make friends with the staff and made sure I learned the names of all the technicians. After all, I was going to be spending a good part of the next seven weeks in their hands. I also had lots of questions these folks might have the answers to. Although I didn't plan it this way, I now realize a part of me was attempting to humanize my situation by connecting with them through an open and friendly demeanor. Okay, I admit that sounds like BS and there was indeed a bit of "fake it till you make it" going on from my end. But what else could I do? My life was in their hands with the treatment they planned and administered.

I teetered between confidence and fear of the unknown. Perhaps they would take *really* good care of me if I befriended them and showed my appreciation. Maybe then, they would take even greater care to position my body oh-so-perfectly and make sure with the ultimate precision that the beams would shoot exactly on target. They would not be satisfied with anything but zapping that tumor with surgical precision and lining everything up just right. Of course, now I realize this is their goal with every patient that walks through "the vault." This is their job as clinicians and professionals. And, to be sure, they did right by me. For that, I am grateful and so is my family.

* * * * * * * * *

Every Monday, the techs would double-check all the measurements of the mask and its alignment with the beams. They would confer with each other and make adjustments, if necessary. Lying there prone and worried, however, all the worst possible thoughts and fears would jump through my mind. For example, on one particular Monday, I heard one technician say to another technician, "Move it up just a *smidge*," or "*a hair.*" I was laying there thinking, "*Smidge* is not even a real word. How the heck can you measure a *smidge* so that the radiation beam will know? How can these two communicate this way for my radiation mask?" Of course, I was feeling vulnerable and insecure, and they were just being human. They ultimately got it right, using their own lingo. But to *me*, I wanted actual measurements. I wanted millimeters or micro-millimeters, or whatever is the smallest increment of real, precise, concrete, indisputable, accurate-to-within-one-atom type of measurement.

I guess I just didn't want human beings at that moment—those capable of making mistakes. I wanted perfection in an imperfect world. I lay there feeling uncomfortable for a while about the whole process, but I didn't have any choice or any say in the matter. So, I beckoned the glass-half-full feeling to wash over me. As soon as it did, I resigned my fate into their hands, closed my eyes, and sighed, "Beam me up, Scotty."

* * * * * * * * *

The first of thirty-three treatments began the first week of April 2012. At five days a week for almost seven weeks, it was a full-time job. Making this commitment on a regular basis required forming a routine in order to make it as smooth and effortless as possible, especially for me as I didn't have full mobility in my left side. For this reason, I was suddenly grateful for handicap ramps. It took brain cancer for me to finally realize they're not just for skateboarders. There was a handy ramp leading to the doorway of the clinic, which made getting around with a walker so much easier. Key word: *easier*, not to be confused with *faster*. A walker on a ramp is still tedious and slow.

One day, we spied a crude, old and rickety hospital-property wheelchair in the lobby. Don't you know, we nabbed it on sight. That relic shaved precious time and aggravation from our car-to-door patient transfer. It also allowed Rich and I to feel like Bonnie and Clyde for a fleeting moment of fun. I suppose you could say we'd become "seasoned" by this time, whatever worked or helped, we were all for it. We quickly realized there's nothing embarrassing about making your life a little easier when you're fighting to get your life back.

During some visits, we had to wait a bit before they were ready to begin my treatment. Thankfully, there were some distractions if we didn't remember to bring our own. In one section of the waiting room, there was a bookshelf full of donated books; mostly fiction, mixed in with the occasional biography. Other reading material consisted of promotional drugs by pharmaceutical companies (I was afraid of those), and brochures about local support groups, yoga instruction, and events for the children of cancer patients. A coffee machine beckoned but I refrained, not because I was trying to be healthy and caffeine-free, per se, but mostly because the creamers were full of artificial ingredients and carbs, which I avoided. There was a good-sized fish tank separating the kids' waiting area from the adult-patient waiting area. This was probably an attempt to keep the kids from getting scared of the zombie-like expressions on us adults waiting to get zapped. I was content with CNN always airing on the television set placed above the fish tank, although it wasn't exactly uplifting to listen, with even only half of my attention, to the latest in school shootings and rogue storms.

* * * * * * * * *

Rich and I were both steadfast in our belief that each radiation treatment would shrink the tumor and, in turn, relieve my symptoms. Once snapped into place, I would go off into my own little world of thought and prayer. These sessions lasted less than fifteen minutes. The techs always had their music going and the thought crossed my mind that I should put in a request for my own playlist. Their soundtrack choices would have been great for an outdoor barbecue, but they weren't exactly in sync with my state of mind during treatment. My thoughts were of prayer, so I would try to conjure up images that could lead to some beneficial, spiritual imagery during each treatment.

As it turned out, the music didn't impact my thoughts or my concentration, one way or the other. The machine itself was rather noisy, and gave off a metallic smell, so I began to mentally incorporate the pings and clangs into a satisfying visual of the tumor slowing eroding and finally surrendering, with a violent death throe, before turning into a cloud of harmless dust.

* * * * * * * * *

Once a week after radiation, I would see the radiation oncologist. We really liked her and we "clicked" right away. Despite my fondness for her and her staff, however, the anticipation of what she would say to us was always stressful. Dr. Katherine McBride, a petite, Asian lady armed with high heels and a huge diamond ring, had a full repertoire of the knowledge I needed for my treatment, but it was knowledge I didn't necessarily want to hear—at least, not yet. Rich asked most of the questions: What clinical trials are available?

How does this work? What if it doesn't? What are our other options? Should we get a second opinion?

At times, I would look at the floor and only take occasional peeks to gauge her expression and body language. My mind was overwhelmed with information and, very likely, tired from radiation. Not sure if I was grasping it all, I secretly hoped Rich could repeat the meat of her answers back to me during the ride home. What I *did* hear was not helpful to my tired mind. She said things like, "You've got a long road ahead of you," and "This is not going to be easy," and (please, not the hair topic), "You'll probably lose your hair." And, finally, this: "This tumor is not a good one." *No shit?* A vivid image that I was disappearing, right then and there, nagged at me. I could feel myself losing grip of my own body. How could I possibly shake myself out of this trance; this feeling that I was being forced out of my own life? I needed to cling to something, but what?

During the first month of treatment, she mentioned to Rich more than to me, something about ash-like material in my brain, a result of the radiation treatments. By this time, the combined words "radiation treatment" seemed like quite the oxymoron. I kept thinking, "What's all this about ash?" I pictured charcoal briquettes decomposing at the bottom of a greasy barbecue pit, ready to fall apart at the first gentle poke of a skewer tip. Was this what that "ash" would look like? Is the radiation making this tumor stuff break down into a gray-black powder in my skull?

I tried to read Dr. McBride's face. Instead, I studied her wedding ring; it was huge. *Business must be good.* Then, I studied her legs. *Maybe she's a runner?* I couldn't help but realize how fortunate she was—she didn't have cancer. As much as I tried to keep my gaze on the doc, I found myself looking at the floor or my fingernails. I had drained my water bottle and now I was getting irritated by the fact that there were no recycling baskets nearby.

By this time, I must have been reflecting the puny persona Rich and Doc McBride must have seen in me, based on their condescending glances. They carried on as if I was a kid sometimes, as if the conversation was way over my head, or I was completely invisible. To be fair, I knew Rich wasn't excluding me from the discussion on purpose. His goal was to make the most of our time with her and ask all of our questions with business-like professionalism, careful to not leave anything out. His goal was to end the meetings with a feeling of empowerment, for both of us, with a feeling like we had a plan B.

As the weeks went by, I would proudly display my latest accomplishments to Doc McBride. The neurological exam was always the same. "Squeeze my thumbs. Push up on my arms. Now push down." With Doc's hand on my knee, "Push my hand up now." "Hold your hands up like you're carrying a pizza. Now, close your eyes. Touch your nose with this finger. Now do that with your right index finger. Walk in a straight line, heel to toe. What's today's date? Where are you? Who's the president? Spell 'world' backwards."

That last one was tough. But I got it right.

CHAPTER 12

BONDING WITH THE ALIEN:
THE NEW YOU

By this time in my journey, I had undergone a needle biopsy surgery, adopted the ketogenic diet (more on this in Part II), and was midway through thirty-three radiation treatments with simultaneous chemotherapy, administered orally. As I said in earlier chapters, the tumor had already caused changes to my physical being even before I knew it was there. The cumulative effect of physical debilitation from the tumor plus the onset of side effects from the cancer treatments made me feel like an alien in my own body. Each day had its ups and downs. I'd like to say the high points more than made up for the low points but that would be a lie. It was like wading into the ocean in between waves, making great progress until one incoming whopper caught you flat-footed and knocked you right back to the sand. Do this a few times and you realize it's exhausting—to the point where it feels futile to make another attempt.

In the beginning, my optimism was in ample supply but my body's physical shortcomings were frustrating and rehabilitation of motor movement wasn't progressing fast enough for my liking.

Balancing a positive mental state in a body that wasn't cooperating made some days harder than others. I latched onto the high points for as long as I could. Sometimes my imagination kicked in and exaggerated my forward progress. I suppose my mind was in self-preservation mode, becoming a cheerleader for my body, which was still playing catch-up. I remember when the radiation techs at the clinic took notice of the progress I was making. When I look back on that moment now, I wonder if they might have overstated my improvement just to build me up psychologically. But at the time, I told myself they had surely seen multiple examples of patients go through all stages of recovery and my progress must have been so exceptional it called for a round of applause. I set myself up to hear more commentary to that effect but I didn't. That's probably because my momentum was moving along exactly as expected—no need to call the Guinness World Record guys. I suppose there comes a point where even radiation techs have to be careful not to build a patient's hopes too high. Nothing is really guaranteed when it comes to cancer treatment. In any case, I hope they realize how much their encouragement meant to me.

One of the most dreaded low points was the nausea and vomiting caused by chemo drugs. I lost count of how many people asked if I was experiencing this. But it's not as big an issue as it used to be, at least from my experience, as well as other patients I came across during treatments. There are many drugs now that combat chemo nausea very effectively, Ondansetron being the wonder drug of the moment. I was given a dose thirty minutes prior to the chemo pills and it worked like a charm. In fact, what hit me worse than anything digestive was the combination of overwhelming exhaustion, loss of appetite, and general malaise. I remember an overall feeling of being unwell, with aches both inside and out. The constant joint and muscle pain sure made it difficult to get anywhere in a hurry. It also added to my feelings of exhaustion because every movement seemed like a battle between mind and body.

* * * * * * * * *

Do you remember being a child and suffering from the flu or bronchitis, something miserable and hard to shake? I do. I would lie there for what seemed an eternity trying to remember what it was like to feel normal, jump out of bed and go play with my friends. During the height of all these treatments, those recollections came back. I couldn't conjure up my old self, the one that was active, vibrant, quick on my feet, well coordinated, and as active as I used to be. That person now seemed like a distant relative, certainly not me.

For example, when I was getting dressed during those seven weeks of radiation, I'd feel the strangest sensation, what seemed like an electrical charge being emitted from my body, something as light as the simple touch of a shirt, as I was putting my arms through the sleeves, would cause this indescribably weird feeling. It was an irritating and frustrating reminder of what my body was being subjected to. I hated the sensation and was relieved when it went away. I believe it was directly related to the radiation I was receiving. How ironic to put such a burden on your body just so it could keep you alive…

Another alien by-product of cancer, due to my left-side weakness, was a new aversion to talking on the phone. Always having held the phone to my left ear, this was now a problem. It was just too weird holding it on the right, and I'd do that until I felt the urge to switch. I'd be chatting it up and the phone would just fall. It would start slipping down my face, right out of my hand. At the same time, speaking itself was no treat due to my mouth being a bit crooked and speech sometimes sounding slurred. Remedies for this were the speakerphone and brief conversations with an apology, as well as communicating through Facebook and text messages. Writing was still difficult, no matter how hard I tried.

Holding a cup or glass was a potential accident. Having dropped more than a couple of items, I played it safe and gave my right hand a few turns. Keeping on with strength training was crucial. Little, silly exercises helped me to believe I could continually re-pave those pathways in the brain. Thoughts of coming out of a coma or learning to walk after an accident came to mind. Many times, I had seen examples of people beating the odds on shows like 60 minutes, 20/20, etc., and here was my very own chance. I now knew firsthand of the burn to come back.

All these alien curiosities did nothing but propel my already unhinged emotions further down into darkness. I hosted pity parties for one every morning while I simultaneously cursed my left side for not cooperating as I struggled to put on my shoes and then tie the laces. Flip-flops would have been great but, unfortunately, when you don't have control of one foot, the flip-flops keep flip-flopping off. Secure shoes were a must and I opted to struggle independently and try tying my own laces rather than ask for too much help. This was certainly a low point.

Sometimes I would scream internally, other times I would scream as loud as I could while in the shower. The frustrations would usually explode when I was in these intimate surroundings. This was where I was most reminded about what normal used to be: surrounded by all my once-special things, taunted by the clothes, shoes and accessories in my closet, lying behind an invisible barrier that I couldn't penetrate in my current state. The alien-me had no need for material things and niceties. But the real me didn't want to let go of them. I began wondering to whom I could pass my special things. The real me knew what that represented and protested by screaming to get out.

These episodes would become a part of my morning ritual. They would subside by the time I was finally dressed and ready to shuffle off to my next treatment or doctor's appointment. I would find my composure and move on with my day as best I could. But I'll never forget, or truly be able to put into words, the deep and sharp despair that echoed in that shower and closet. It didn't help that I also sensed my explosions of grief were unfair to my husband. The last thing I intended to do was start our day with such a negative state of mind. But that's cancer. It tries to bring you to your knees. The emotional pain is real and it's okay to let it out. I tried to not point it in anyone's direction. But I had to let off some steam when I was alone. When I did, I found my calm shortly after. This phase didn't last too long, thankfully.

The absence of one particular symptom took me by surprise. You would think someone with a brain tumor would experience frequent headaches. I certainly had a few, especially right around the time of my diagnosis, but it wasn't a constant and overwhelming problem. Even after my surgery, I rarely experienced headaches. I'm very thankful for that. If I was getting severe and constant headaches on top of everything else I was feeling, I would be wondering if the tumor was growing. We would all be assuming things were getting worse, or entertaining the formation of a dreaded blood clot.

Knowing you have a tumor in your brain is like knowing you have a parasite living inside your body. That's what cancer is. It's an unwelcome invader and your body is its host. It will ravage you if it can. I might have entertained myself with pity parties for a while there, but I was growing tired of this alien version of myself. My anger was starting to awaken. This was a good sign. My spirited self was trying to make a comeback. But it couldn't come fast enough.

With all the limitations I was feeling, it became almost like a game for me to focus on what control I did have over my body and my mind. I was able to sleep well and I'm sure that helped regenerate my weary body overnight. I didn't experience any visual or auditory problems but, as I said, I suddenly had a mid-Western accent, caused by the weakness along my entire left side, from my face down the whole length of my body. It was interesting that I was still able to concentrate on a specific task and stick with it for a decent chunk of time. At least I had some control.

I tried to remind myself of these positives. It wasn't easy but every positive can be reinforced and, as the treatments hopefully go to work on the cancer, the alien-you may take a back seat to the real you.

It takes time and faith, that's all true, but any progress going forward should be applauded and noted. Use each milestone as ammunition in your will to defy and conquer your disease, chin-up, with attitude. Make a stand against whatever waves of resistance remain. By the time your treatments are done, your test results may embolden you to feel the same momentum of hope that I did. But, again, there are no guarantees against the monster called Cancer.

These ups and downs will be different for everyone, but the emotional impact may be the same. Cancer is such a personal disease. No matter how many people we know who have it, it's more likely than not that each of those people reacts to it differently. Sometimes I let the lows knock me down. After a few times on the ground, however, I'm the kind that gets truly pissed off and fights to stay up the next time. It's good to let your inner pit bull rise up and tell cancer where to go. This isn't a time to be bashful. Let it all out. After all, you're fighting for your life.

This quote by Dante, Italian philosopher and poet, sums up my feelings:

"There is no greater sorrow than to recall happiness in times of misery."
Dante Allighieri

* * * * * * * * *

The topic of hair loss always seems to be one of great concern to a newly diagnosed cancer patient, for good reason. Many chemotherapy treatment regimens lead to some level of hair loss. When I was first diagnosed, I remember sitting in the neuro-oncologist's office and feeling the gravity of my diagnosis sinking in. Hair loss was the farthest thing from my mind, a big zero. Dr. Patchell started going on about hair trivia. "Some people don't lose much." "For some, it grows back a different color, or not at all." My response went something like this: "Please just stop. I couldn't care less about what happens on the outside of my head. Can we get back to what really matters—that thing *inside* my head?" Of course he knew all that really mattered was what we were going to do about this beast in my brain. He was merely trying to prepare me for the inevitable question most people in my position would have: "When will all my hair fall out?" I couldn't care less about hair. I preferred to not waste time on the topic.

Here's what did happen with my hair: I didn't lose any of it until halfway through the thirty-three radiation treatments. This somehow felt like a small victory—as if I had anything to do with it. It began slowly. I started noticing stray hairs on my pillow, some in the sink, and lots in my hairbrush. None of this disturbed me since I was expecting it. I was even curious about shaving it off. I wondered how that would feel and look. I suppose that sounds odd. It was kind of interesting, in a twisted way, when I ran my fingers through my hair and pulled out large sections. I remember riding in the car with the window down and I would just release the hairs into the air. In a way, it was liberating. When enough hair fell out, Rich and I decided it was time to shave it all off. I also remember laughing to myself as I pictured people on the sidewalk doing double takes at the sight of hair tufts floating behind our car as I tossed out what was between my fingers.

There were a handful of people who had pledged to shave their heads as a gesture of unity and support. But that didn't happen and that was okay with me. I was always uncomfortable with that idea. I know people mean well but I just don't see the necessity of such an act, although I can understand if, for example, a parent did it to support their child. But for me, the act itself wouldn't actually accomplish anything. I would still have brain cancer, and no hair. Another reason why I'm glad it didn't happen is that I didn't want to worry about somebody feeling resentful, or having regrets and then possibly unloading on me.

To be honest, I didn't mind being bald. It was a major time-saver in the morning. My hair actually grew back quickly and I had to trim it often and be creative with hair accessories to keep it off my face when it was in that in-between phase. To my surprise, it grew back curly and dark, with no gray. I never did lose my eyelashes or brows. I wouldn't have minded losing hair on the parts that require shaving, but I wasn't that lucky.

Of course, everyone will experience baldness differently. I wasn't uncomfortable being bald. It was during this time that I found Angelique White, a photographer in my area who offers her services complimentary to cancer patients like myself in order to do her *Bald Is Beautiful* series. It was empowering and I'm proud of all the photos she did for me.

＊＊＊＊＊＊＊＊＊

The lighter side of bonding with the alien-you borne from cancer is looking at the bright side, which includes all the preferential treatment that comes to those viewed as invalids, or those not long for this world. I don't say this to be flippant about my disease (no one knows more deeply than I do that there's nothing frivolous about battling cancer), but the bright spots during this scary journey are so few and far between, finding any comedy or levity along the way adds a valuable gift: that wonderful little thing called a "smile."

Think of it as "pulling the Cancer card." The truth is, when we're healthy and vibrant, more often than not we find those around us too busy to stop what they're doing and help, or even ask if we need help. If you're like I was before cancer, a dynamo that never stopped and always had it under control, everyone assumes, "You got this." Now, here I come, the Energizer Bunny without the batteries, plodding along with the help of a walker, not a drum, a bald beacon of skull instead of the sunglasses, all of the above alerting those around me to my sad situation. People, even strangers, would stop what they were doing and offer all kinds of wonderful accommodations.

Restaurants will be happy to adjust the thermostat to whatever temperature makes you comfortable, other diners be damned. You want to order from the children's menu? Go for it. If you're a woman, you'll have a much better chance of getting someone to offer you his or her seat on public transportation while sporting a bald scalp rather than a pregnant belly. Waiting in line will become a thing of the past: you'll be ushered to the front at almost any venue. Have you ever dropped something near others and realized no one was going to bend over to pick it up for you? Well, fear no more. Drop everything you like, sit back, and enjoy the tug-of-war that ensues. Eager helpers will materialize out of the woodwork to snatch whatever you dropped off the ground before you can blurt, "Help!" If you can drive while you're bald, you'll find you may as well be driving a police cruiser; that's how immune you'll be from law enforcement finding a minor reason to stop and question your abilities. The same goes for minor parking lot infractions. Those dents and fender-benders you caused? They're nothing to be concerned about. No one wants to take the insurance money of a dying cancer patient. In fact, everyone who encounters your presence will offer you a smile, even those who have been waiting a half an hour because you're late, because, hey, you have cancer, you have a right to be late now. Are you unwilling to pretend you like someone else's home-cooking? Simply tell them you're nauseous from chemo. No one will doubt you. You are free. Well, except for that parasite in your body...

I really enjoyed the time Rich and I went away for a Mexican holiday while I was sporting my baldness. As I was limping along the customs line, someone called for a wheelchair and whisked us to the front of the line. Yes, in this case, some had a hissy fit but were quickly shamed into submission by others around them who, surprise, smiled congenially.

Disclaimer: These snippets are recounted in jest. I never overstepped my boundaries, put anyone in harm's way or drove like a banshee. There were serious shortcomings in my abilities to walk, stand, eat, etc. If ever there was one surprisingly bright spot to illuminate my cancer journey, it was the kindness of strangers. I never took it for granted. The pay-it-forward mentality of most people, when faced with another's obvious suffering from a deadly disease, restored my faith in humanity. It may do the same for you, if you're ever faced with such an ordeal.

* * * * * * * * *

Before my diagnosis, sleep was rarely an issue for me. I had insomnia now and then, or maybe interrupted sleep, after which I lay awake no matter how hard I tried to fall back into slumber. But the old me had no real issue with a lack of rest. When I was healthy, my sleep clock was programmed for evenings only. That all changed with the onset of astrocytoma. The growing tumor, the swelling it caused in my brain, and all the meds and radiation took a toll on my energy level. The new alien-me needed naps on a regular basis, no matter what time of day it was. I found it effortless to relax and quickly fall asleep, in spite of any background or household noise. This was a real benefit during my treatments. Each nap break allowed me to recharge enough to move on to the next appointment or task. Daytime snoozes for the old me would only happen when I was sick, and that was rare.

I was constantly reminded by the professionals to rest when my body demanded it. Wanting to be a good patient, I took heed and found it very beneficial for both my body and my mind. The body needs rest in order to fight the cancer—and deal with all the radiation and chemo drugs, which are so harsh on the system. It didn't take long for me to realize there's no sense in fighting the urge to rest or sleep. It doesn't do any good to push your body and risk the effectiveness of your treatments. In my case, I didn't have a whole lot stopping me from daytime napping. The kids were in school. Rich was working from home. We had relatives rotating in and out of town. Friends and neighbors were making us dinner. So I was a good patient, and good to my body. I slept.

* * * * * * * * *

One thing I noticed, which was very cool and never happened before my diagnosis, was feeling totally detached from time. The alien me would doze off without a care, in whatever quiet spot it could find, and enter a REM sleep so quickly that my body recharged quicker than a redlined iPhone. Old-me was jealous of alien-me on this point—how super efficient to feel so good so fast! I remember waking up from one of these power naps and thinking that hours had gone by but it was only twenty minutes, and I felt completely rejuvenated. My body was on autopilot.

In spite of all these regular daytime snoozes, I still found myself needing sleep every night, and it came quickly. Even if I woke up in the middle of the night to use the bathroom, I would go right back to bed and glide into dreamland. All of this rest meant my moods were generally good when I opened my eyes each new day. Over time, every morning became a blessing. I was traveling further down the road to recovery and my body felt like it was regrouping. More and more, I found myself thanking God for the rest I had just experienced, and for all my family's blessings.

* * * * * * * * *

I find it interesting that my dreams were positive, in spite of my condition. This could be attributed to my faith in God and how this faith allowed me to let go, somewhat. I suppose those who don't believe in God could also find that peace, if they have enough faith in themselves as fighters, able to somehow win the battle against cancer—or, at the very least, to accept whatever fate lies in their future with some semblance of peace. Either way, it's certainly not easy. When I found myself pushed into a corner, facing this beast called cancer, I started playing life on a new game board. Just as all human beings are resilient, I learned new tricks and new strategies. It's not like I had a choice, but if you have a family, it would be very selfish to just give up and wait to die.

Once Rich and I settled into our new routine (five days a week of radiation therapy and clinical visits for a full seven week stretch), and we could see that rest could be had in spite of this ordeal, the peace we experienced during these quiet moments was blissful. The breaks we programmed into our days allowed us both to regroup from the physical and mental strains we were each burdened with.

Our bedroom became our haven. Lying down comfortably became the perfect set-up for moments of prayer, which we also found soothing. It helped to have an uncluttered bedroom, a new set of sheets, and a pretty bed-set (a thoughtful gift from Rich's mom). Every morning, I would remove the remnants of sleep to make the bed pristine, anticipating coming home from the radiation clinic to our little slice of heaven. Our bedroom has a view of central Arizona's White Tank Mountains and our backyard pool. At night, the pool lights would glow softly and I could hear the wind rustling through the fronds of the palm trees. Wind chimes would sing their song gently along the fence. Day or night, the conditions were just right for recharging.

CHAPTER 13

SPIRITUALITY AND OUTLOOK

Joy: The emotion of great delight, or happiness, caused by something exceptionally good or satisfying; keen pleasure; elation. Joy is the deeper version of happiness, the kind that comes from within, and it can be experienced even during difficult circumstances.

For me, discovering joy and understanding it's true meaning was especially important throughout my journey. I learned it was much more than fleeting moments of happiness, or just an over-used word in a Christmas card. While fighting cancer, I discovered it's possible to be scared and joyful at the same time. It's a spiritual calmness that takes little effort, if you allow yourself to welcome its embrace.

Think of it this way: you've been told by a reliable source that you will enjoy life on this planet for only a short time longer. What would you do? There are a couple of options to this dilemma. One option is you could shut down, turn inward and cease all meaningful contributions to Mother Earth and humanity. Another option is to willfully experience a super-concentrated love for your family and all those you hold dear—and more than ever, now, because you know you'll be leaving them soon, forever.

If you choose the latter, gratitude and hope, rather than the former, bitterness and surrender, you may see what I've seen: the world through a lens of divine clarity. Everything around me was outlined with a sharpness I never noticed before. I saw even ordinary, everyday things as if I was seeing them for the first time, because I was keenly aware the day would soon come when I wouldn't see them again.

If you're like me, you may even see things that never stood out before, those things you used to take for granted. The spiritual side of the reality that surrounds you may let you know you've been too busy to grasp it all because you took it for granted. You were in a happy-go-lucky, pre-cancer state of mind. Once I opened my eyes, this incredible revelation resulted in all things trivial being shed like an unwanted skin. I vowed to never again spend time on the frivolous and the superficial. It was a spiritual transformation that bordered on magic. The great news is, once you feel this like I have, you can live the rest of your life with the freedom of feeling grounded in what truly matters in life: the intangibles and those you love.

* * * * * * * * *

Looking at life through a new lens framed by mortality, I learned to stop wasting my time on foolishness. Those who spent their days filling the air with gossip and critical commentary about others would soon become targets of my persuasion to steer the conversation toward a topic of substance. If you're in my shoes, facing a physical battle with cancer, don't neglect the fact that you also need mental and emotional medicine. Toxic people should have no place in your life. As you make your best attempt to purge your body of disease, try your best to also purge your universe from negativity.

If you're religious or at all spiritual, this is a good time to dive deeper into your faith. I find tremendous comfort in group prayer and helping others as much as I can. Allowing your spiritual side to grow, especially during trying times like cancer battles, will improve your outlook and help your healing process, physically and mentally. It will put your situation in perspective. This doesn't mean the struggles we face become any less significant; *it reminds us we aren't lone sufferers in this world.* I'm not the first person with terminal brain cancer, and I certainly won't be the last. Almost everyone I know knows someone who either has, had, or died from cancer already. In the scheme of things, none of us really stands out. But we can try to help others through our own ordeal. Writing this book is my contribution; making the best of my experience in order to help others learn something from cancer rather than just give up and give in to its deadly mystery, becoming just another one of its victims.

I wish I didn't have cancer. But knowing there are many cancer patients who face it without family or loved ones reminds me to appreciate the support I *do* have, in spite of why I need it. I don't have time to be bitter and question the "Why's." I'd rather move beyond that negativity and be grateful for not being alone, and for whatever time I have left. The more I see and help others in need, the better I feel about myself—cancer be damned.

* * * * * * * * *

This leads me to a big issue facing those with life-threatening diseases: questioning our own self-worth within society, especially in such an incapacitated state, dealing with tumor growth and cancer treatments. My self worth deteriorated quickly. I had to stop working because of the rapid onset of partial, stroke-like paralysis in the entire left side of my body. The sting was rather harsh because I had just remodeled an office for my life-coaching business and the ink on my business cards was barely dry. Just two or three weeks into my venture, the symptoms began. I swear I can still hear the loud, sucking sound of my dreams being deflated, like a beautiful balloon that got away.

Without a purpose, and now quite helpless, I immediately felt like a burden. Suddenly, I was dependent on others all the time. My self-worth turned into, "What self-worth?" "What was the point in maintaining me," was a question I remember asking myself after my needle biopsy surgery, when I didn't think I would survive. After all, at that time, it was just a matter of weeks from the time I was normal to when I was suddenly speaking with a mysterious Michigan accent, unable to either write or walk without assistance. This transition was so abrupt it made me wonder if I would ever be *me* again. It also made me wonder if I was worth all the time people were wasting on me.

****

The joy concept I talked about earlier would not be immediate; it would only emerge after several difficult but key triumphs, and only after I began to put into practice a sincere desire to make whatever time I had left with my husband and children full of love and quality. There was little room for anything else. I'm thankful my faith continued to grow, to the point where it finally sunk in that even in a different condition, I remained me and I was valuable and worth saving.

It's a shame this kind of validation and prioritization too often comes about after we're pushed into a corner. I've heard people talk about how prisoners "find God." Rich and I already had a firm foundation; both of us were raised Roman Catholic and we'd completed all the sacraments. Even so, we were surprised to find how much our faith grew since my diagnosis. Another surprise was to see this happening to our children as well.

Within our church, a group called "Summit Sisters" was formed. One of the leaders shared with me a series of topics that would be featured over the upcoming months. I was asked to speak about inspiration. This was an honor I didn't expect so I got busy planning what I would say. The end result was sharing the life-changing event of my cancer diagnosis, important milestones that followed, and whatever highlights gave me hope. It was important for me to emphasize how I was still able to feel happy despite having cancer, through the growth in my faith and the support of my dear family and friends.

Sharing my struggle and its undercurrent of acceptance through faith was itself rewarding to me, but another silver lining from participating in this event was how it brought me closer to many members of our church. This motivated me to get even more involved with their outreach, so I began doing some volunteer work. It was gratifying and I really enjoyed the interaction. I visited the church office once a week, made phone calls, and wrote letters to new members or people suffering from difficulty. Touching someone else's life was very fulfilling, and this happened even if they didn't know me. These positive vibes began to morph into the reason why I decided to write this book. Why not chronicle my journey? If just one cancer patient could find solace in my words and validation of their fears and struggles, I could embolden another life against the paralyzing power of cancer.

Through a newly formed network of church members who attended the outreach, the idea blossomed to host a growth group for women at my home. Rich and I had hosted a similar event a year before for couples only, but this was different. This particular group brought me closer to some ladies I otherwise would not have come to know. Our Christian faith was a solid basis for growing friendships through our common goal of deepening our faith. The benefits from this enhanced my personal life with another layer of calm to help me weather the storm of my disease.

I think it's interesting to look back at my spiritual progress over the first year of my physical battle with cancer. My Caring Bridge site was set up on March 1, 2012, in preparation for a series of initial tests and procedures. This site would become my one-stop communication hub to let friends and family know what was going on from that point on, and how to help if necessary, without us having to call, email or text people.

The thoughts in my mind following the initial shock of my diagnosis were dark, full of fear and worry. Reading this early Caring Bridge entry shows how much spiritual strength I experienced throughout that first year. It changed my entire outlook on life. We've since taken down the Caring Bridge site because my condition has since stabilized and we're past the need to broadcast updates. In any event, here's that post:

Caring Bridge Blog Entry, March 23, 2013, 11:43 pm:

About a year ago:
...I was given the worst news of my life.
...I was stunned and afraid.
...I started losing control of many everyday functions.
...my family started losing control.
...my peer group consisted of sick, declining people using canes, walkers and wheelchairs.
...I didn't think I should obtain or be given anything new because I wouldn't be around to use it.
...I decided to fight. To fight hard.
...I started searching, seeking, meditating, discovering.
...I started to sort things out.
...I began to realize I had some practical survival skills that others could also be applying, regardless of disease or perceived/assumed health.
...I slowly I woke up.
...My life started to become better.

* * * * * * * * *

Another extreme low that can cloud your outlook and be sparked by any number of catalysts, is mourning for your life, and mourning the loss of who you were before cancer. This new me that I jokingly call "alien-me" in the previous chapter, is real and a force to be reckoned with. The reality of its existence started a tidal wave of deep longing for my old body and its functionality. It almost felt as if the old me died and I was grieving its loss. The usual emotions piled on, anger, frustration, self-pity, in one word, bitterness.

I wish I could say there's a remedy for this phase but it's deeply personal and any progress you make to overcome it will only come at your own pace. All I can say is that it's possible. I alluded to this earlier, but it bears repeating: the path toward pushing past this period requires you to meet it head-on, confront it, and have the fortitude to see any silver linings beyond it on the horizon. No, you will most likely never, ever be the same person you were before cancer (both mentally and physically). But you may experience physical improvements as your treatments take hold, and you may also experience gratification from an outpouring of support from those around you. This could be enough to help you down the path of confronting the negativity in your mind and replacing it with a positive outlook that could, in turn, help you heal physically.

Early on, I may have wanted to hit someone who told me, "Don't worry. Your life will ultimately be better for having this disease." Well, don't shoot the messenger, but it's true. Of course, that's because I'm surviving.

If you're playing the game of life and death at all, you should be playing to win your life back. If you accept death, you're not competing in a game, you've already forfeited. These passages will fall on deaf ears to those who feel that way. It's unfortunate. But I'm not here to persuade or to evangelize, only to share my struggle and offer hope to those willing to add ammunition to their own battle against cancer.

* * * * * * * * *

As important as it was for my own spirituality and outlook to be healthy and elevated by those around me, I also realized the importance of those closest to me having a healthy attitude as well, my husband and children, in particular. Seeing me suffering without any guarantees my life would be saved wore them down. Elevating my own outlook started a positive domino effect on them. But even before I was fully positive, they took the initiative to rally support and boost my spirits. It's a tender gesture, being a cheerleader for a cause you can't predict. It's evident to me now though, when it's someone you love, such as a spouse, parent or child, friends and family often feel a sense of helplessness and this is combined with a touch of guilt for not having cancer themselves.

The attempt from my family to rally others early on started when Rich decided to order a few-hundred rubber bracelets with a customized message to support me. He seemed to enjoy even the quest itself, searching for the quickest processing at the best price, which varies depending on the number of characters you want printed on the bracelets, and by the quantity. We chose the color gray, imprinted with my name and the word "endurance," which is also what the newly acquired Asian tattoo on my back means. The clincher for Rich was a special deal: *BUY 200, GET 200 FREE!* or something to that effect. We passed them out liberally to our friends at church and to our kids' classmates and teammates at school. When we traveled east to visit family, we piled a bunch on the table, free for the taking. It always warms my heart to see these bracelets being worn, especially after so many months have passed.

T-shirts are a popular support symbol also. At a fund-raiser held for our family, the team of friends who ran the day's events all sported T-shirts with *Team Mindy* inscribed on the front and this Bible quote on the back: *Watch, stand fast in the faith, be brave, be strong. Let all that you do be done with love. — 1 Corinthians 16:13-14*

After seeing these rally trinkets, T-shirts and events, it really hit home that cancer affects those around the patient much more than this patient could ever have imagined. It's another reason why I choose to be positive and look for the bright spot that goes even beyond my own recovery. That's not easy, especially in the beginning of the recovery journey. At first glance, you might think, "How selfless," and "How unrealistic." I can tell you from experience that it's neither. What it *is* is a release, a pure and unadulterated release.

TIP: While your caregiver is trying to shield you from everyday life issues, the pressure of maintaining a game face while watching cancer take its toll on you can be overwhelming. Don't take it personally if a caregiver has an occasional meltdown. It's not you. It's the cancer and the pressures of life without you. Let them vent and try to discuss solutions after the emotions dissipate.

---

* * * * * * * * *

The glare of cancer is a spotlight that shines a little too bright for me. From the minute I learned about the astrocytoma in my brain, I became the center of unwanted attention. My physical disabilities, even before we knew their source, began an onslaught of speculation about my condition that made me uncomfortable and self-conscious. It was actually a relief for me to begin considering others for a change, and shift the focus elsewhere when possible. Of course, when you have cancer those around you will never forget that you are the center of attention. But I learned one way to spread the spotlight was to be inclusive and let those around me help us in whatever capacity was necessary at the moment, and also let them do their support rallies.

We started our home headquarters, nicknamed "Camp Onion," the brainchild of a dear friend who happened to be at our house with his wife and kids when my neurologist friend, Troy, came by to reveal the first MRI results. When Troy said my tumor was the size of an onion, my first response was the horror of the difference sizes of onions. So, I shot back, "What *kind* of onion are we talking here, scallion, shallot, Vidalia, Maui?" Everyone who heard me broke out in laughter and the name of our headquarters stuck.

Camp Onion was where friends would convene, dry erase pens in hand, ready to mark up white boards and calendars listing out a schedule of events to help us out. We planned out rides to appointments, meal deliveries, and listed our friends' phone numbers and our kids' closest friends information as well, just in case a distraction or extra help was necessary if I had to suddenly be hospitalized. A lot of this information was transferred to our Caring Bridge website, so everyone who logged on could be on the same page. This was a great start toward inclusiveness and helped alleviate some of our stress, although it also introduced a different kind of dilemma.

The meal mission was intense and having people in our home for various chores was a little difficult to get used to. In the beginning of our new cancer life, there were awkward moments when the five-o'clock-hour approached (someone decided five o'clock was a good time for people to bring a meal by). Of course, that was fine and well intentioned, being early enough for us to have dinner ready for the kids and early enough for those delivering the meal to get back home in time for their own dinner. I, for one, didn't have plans at that time of day. I was usually wiped out from radiation and chemo. Rich and I could check the Caring Bridge website to see what was being brought and by whom. Depending on my level of fatigue (or despair) at the appointed hour, I would decide whether I was up to exchanging pleasantries and say, "Thank you," or in the dumps and hide in my room, instead.

This sounds really great, and it is, but it's not always easy to be inclusive. It's worth it, though, because allowing others to chip in was best for my family. It also reminded me that cancer is a selfish disease and that I should fight it in the most unselfish of ways. Let everyone into your battle! Yes, it's about you, but it's also about them. Let them help you. The more ammunition you have to fight cancer, the better off you are. It's a great life lesson, and one of the silver linings of this horrible disease.

CHAPTER 14

INTIMACY AND SELF-CONFIDENCE

This is a topic rarely covered in cancer books. That's probably because both the cancer patient and the intimate partner are reluctant to discuss physical gratification when one of the two is fighting just to survive. Many of the common side effects from chemotherapy include nausea and fatigue so great, the last thing on a patient's mind is sex or intimacy. Most partners wouldn't encroach on this subject for fear of being selfish.

I can say with honesty that cancer does its best to rob a woman of her sexiness. It's hard to emulate a goddess when you can't speak properly, or move half your body without great effort and awkwardness. But on the other hand, you can only hope your partner sees beyond the image of you that cancer has created; that he or she still remembers the you *before* cancer, the one that enjoyed moments of intimacy or passion. The insecurity that comes with cancer and its treatments were unavoidable for me; I'm sure they are for most others, as well.

It's almost as if a person becomes asexual when in treatment. It's just not possible to function the same and feel the same subtle tingles of warmth and excitement. It almost seems like those parts are broken, or they simply got "turned off," were put on "idle," and you hope, one day, after cancer, they'll resume their normal functions with the same vigor and effectiveness as before. I've heard, for some, it's never the same, for a variety of reasons. What a shame. It's just another aspect of life that cancer can destroy.

For all these reasons, intimacy and closeness tend to be avoided during treatment. But, as I said, it doesn't mean that intimacy isn't wanted or needed from a cancer patient, or from a partner for that matter. For some partners who don't push the issue, or even bring it up, there may be a fear of hurting something. Mix this fear with all the outward side effects a patient may display, and it certainly makes sense that sex and intimacy wouldn't be at the forefront of a partner's mind. These become luxuries to hope for in the months ahead, they take a backseat to the more important things, such as rest, medication and recovery. Also, life is hectic during a cancer treatment plan. In our case, add three kids and you can imagine the last thing on our minds was intimacy. But intimacy remains crucial to the well being between couples.

Throughout this book I've been careful not to seem as if I'm giving advice rather than suggestions from first-hand experience, but in this area, I'm going to go with my instincts. Even if you don't have the desire or the energy, your partner may need you, and you probably need your partner too. I believe any level of intimacy is better than none. If you can hold each other, or at least have parts of your bodies touch, the skin contact will help nourish your relationship.

We live in Arizona, where it's hot most of the time and, therefore, very natural to sleep with few or no clothes on. Just giving in to this simple practice of sleeping with little or no clothing can begin to melt away any caregiver/patient roles. It's possible this might spark a little of that once-common intimacy, and remind you of the couple you once were. It's a wonderful feeling to realize, "Yes, we still exist, that couple in love before cancer tried to come in between us."

Depending on your condition, getting into an intimate, yet comfortable, position of relaxation and pleasure may involve some creativity, maybe some previously uncharted territory. But it's worth a try. It might take some effort but I strongly urge couples to at least make an attempt to figure out a way (or two or three) that can make both of you happy.

I'm not just talking about sex. By intimacy, I also mean tenderness, which can be extremely deep and satisfying. It can make you both feel like yourselves again by allowing that closeness, that feeling of femininity or masculinity, of being reacquainted with the way you shared private moments, holding each other before cancer, and remembering the things that turned you on. For Rich and me, sharing inside jokes and laughing a lot (at ourselves mostly) helped ease our tension and made us feel normal again. And it made me feel alive.

TIP: Caregivers: Remind yourself that a cancer patient is well aware their body is in battle. The reality that cancer may win and their body may gradually shut down makes mortality an in-your-face fear. Tread lightly on the fragile emotional state of whomever you care for.

TIP: Even during intimate moments, it's easy to get caught up in cancer-themed discussions and nothing else. Try to put cancer talk aside once in a while for an intimate discussion about hope instead. Plan a trip for when your health improves. Keep your dreams alive with something to look forward to after cancer, something to shoot for beyond just the physical battle of everyday treatments.

---

* * * * * * * * *

There are some intimate moments that are anything but sexy, yet they're a necessity. For about a month after my first go-round with the surgeon, the needle biopsy, my motor skills and movements were very restricted and came with much difficulty, mostly on my left side. I was a hazard to myself, what the professionals call a "fall risk." At this point in my cancer journey, Rich needed to help me shower and get dressed.

You may remember, we've been together since college, when we were eighteen years old, and we have no shortage of experiences through all levels of intimacy: sickness, bodily functions, three C-sections (which Rich witnessed), childcare, and deeply passionate love. Rich has seen it all and has done it all with me. He experienced my water break in bed, cleaned me up, and changed my pads while slipping in my blood on the hospital floor after each C-section. We still joke about the first time we experienced meconium shooting out of our firstborn's butt and hitting the wall in the hospital. You get the idea.

In spite of this comfort level, I experienced an increase in stress during this time—a sense of heightened aggravation. Where was this coming from? Needing help taking a shower was not an issue, and being naked was certainly not an issue. I realized it was *helplessness* that was the issue, and a painful one at that. After all, how bizarre to not be able to jump in the shower when the urge hits you? Not knowing if I would be permanently disabled and dependent on others was the real problem—the "stressor," the catalyst for my rage, which began to flare up around this point in my treatment. I couldn't help but wonder if cancer would take away my independence for these very personal but daily rituals forever. It was a rude awakening and I had to keep my rage in check. I called on my faith to help calm my fears. It worked.

Rich remained patient and sweet, in spite of my tantrum moments. He would help me get in the shower and get started with my routine. It was endearing to see him in my closet trying to pick out clothes that matched, and trying to figure out which direction the underwear went, or how to hook the bra. His attentiveness was, quite honestly, adorable. In fact, he was so afraid to walk away from the bathroom while I was in the shower that I had to convince him I wouldn't attempt to get out without him. He was terrified of me falling and banging my head. In general, I was compliant, but I had some moments that led Rich to see a side of my personality he hadn't seen before, and neither had I. But that's cancer for you, full of surprises.

* * * * * * * * *

In the early days of post-surgical recovery, I tended to gravitate toward the most comfortable clothes I could get my hands on, to wear around the house, for naps, or to go out in public. Sweatpants became a necessity at that time but they never made me feel very feminine or attractive. So, gradually, as I was able to break away from them, I started wearing clothing that was both comfortable and attractive, things that made me feel pretty and that I knew Rich liked.

Make-up went by the wayside for a couple of months as well. Before my radiation treatments started, I either read or learned from someone that I shouldn't wear lotions or make up. Generally speaking, nothing should be applied to your skin four hours before your treatment. In any case, it was easier to just go without because putting on make-up, such as mascara, was physically very difficult and frustrating given the loss of grip in my left hand and the fact that I was left-handed. In fact, I passed on make-up for the entire seven weeks of radiation. I have to admit, it was liberating to let it go, but I didn't feel my best. At first, I was too overwhelmed to care. My looks didn't matter much to me at that time. I had more serious issues on my mind than make-up or clothes.

As I started to recover more of my motor functions, especially those in my left hand, I became more capable with it and quickly got back into my normal routine of grooming and dressing. I started putting on mascara and doing things that required dexterity and a steady hand.

* * * * * * * * *

Another source of confidence in the looks department came from the feedback I was getting about my baldness. People told me I pulled it off quite well and many of my friends suggested I try big, hoop earrings and bright lipstick. It was at this time that I found the wonderfully talented photographer, Angelique White, who I introduced earlier and who's acquiring photos of bald cancer patients for a series in her professional portfolio. I signed on for a complimentary photo shoot and she did a beautiful collage that everyone agreed really captured the human strength and dignity patients like me fight so hard to preserve.

While some of these cosmetic touches improved my confidence and my appearance, one thing that never did improve was my gait. I still have some functionality issues on my left side, and a limp. Another repercussion of left-sided weakness is my inability to keep a flip-flop on my left foot for more than a few steps. That's a shame since flip-flops are a basic wardrobe essential in the heat of Arizona for most of the year. This weakness is caused by radiation damage that permanently interrupted some signals from my brain to the rest of my body. This communication gap interferes with my ability to dance, run and walk with the feminine flair I used to have. High heels are definitely out of the question, especially if they don't have a good strap. Although I admit I miss all these things, I'm even more grateful to be able to get up every day and walk to the bathroom on my own. Heck, I'm just thrilled to be alive.

Over time, as my energy levels increased and I got stronger, I became interested in accessorizing again. I pulled out my pretty tops and even started matching outfits to purses and shoes. I was making a come back! This was when I started feeling more like a woman and a wife than a cancer patient. There's nothing wrong with that. If you're inclined to feel better, more like your old self, with pretty things and clothes, go for it. Take it gradually as I did but don't ever feel like the little details don't have the power to make you feel a great deal better about yourself. When you're dealing with cancer, baldness, and a limp, those pretty bangles and beads, that lovely shade of lipstick, could work wonders on your psyche.

Tip: Try to spend quality time with your partner that takes the emphasis off their caregiver role. It's hard to be a couple when cancer is the unwanted third companion, but try to do something outside of doctor's visits, treatment appointments and pharmacy runs. Go on a movie date, hold hands in the park, take a Sunday drive with no destination, just the two of you.

---

* * * * * * * * *

Speaking of psyche, for the first year that my tumor was inoperable, I couldn't help but feel that if it didn't shrink to dust, at some point it might kill me. I wondered what would happen to Rich when I disappeared from this Earth. What will he do? Who will he find? What will she look like?

I wanted to have some conversations with Rich about him getting together with someone else in the future if I passed away. I told him I'd like him to find a maternally inclined, fine, Christian woman. I had it all planned out. Of course, I know that's not how it works in real life. I just wanted him to be happy and not be lonely if I didn't beat this. I knew he would be in for a very tough time.

It was most important to me that there be a woman who could love Rich and our kids as much as I did. Looking back on this now, I realize that was wishful thinking. No one could ever love Rich and my kids that much. In any case, Rich assured me I didn't have to be involved in this area and he would take care of that on his own, if and when it was necessary.

I don't mean to make light of this, or seem stoic about this topic; it's an extremely painful one for me to think about. I suppose I just wanted to give her an orientation to our life and to our stuff, so I can bear some responsibility for making things right when I'm gone, if that were to be the case. On a lighter note, I would like to orient her to all of *my* stuff, and instruct her on how not to mess up the Tupperware. I have a fantastic system in place. She'll need to understand and appreciate that.

In all seriousness, most cancer patients in my shoes may have these thoughts, especially those with young children who are used to a two-parent household. Who will fill the void when you're gone? If someone doesn't, won't the kids suffer? I admit, as easy as it was for me to talk to Rich about it, I was never able to talk to my kids about it. I suppose I just can't go there. A couple of opportunities arose for me to bring up the subject. I told the kids I wanted Daddy to be happy and for the kids to be content with whatever changes take place after I pass. As a family, we've been very honest about my disease. We've made it through some very difficult moments, for over two years now, of trying to put cancer behind us. But the harsh realities they've had to deal with over this time made me hesitant to add anything more to the burden they're facing. It's already been a lifetime's worth.

CHAPTER 15

PERSONAL GROWTH

A whole new set of priorities emerged during my first year of fighting a malignant brain tumor. These resulted in multiple areas of personal growth. As I said in earlier chapters, many were a result of the interactions I had with those around me, specifically, my friends and family. My outward reactions projected a new standard of behavior and acceptance, one that allowed no room for negativity or entertaining anything superficial. In this chapter, I'd like to discuss the deeper growth inside myself, the areas that usually remain private. By sharing the candid emotions and resolutions I had during this trying time, I hope to prove that not only are these feelings normal, given the circumstances, but also that they're healthy and can be stepping stones for a renewed approach to life, one that can sustain you even after cancer, with some priceless personal growth.

One noteworthy milestone for me was relinquishing my fear of how others would judge me, on a variety of levels. Learning to embrace this concept isn't easy and it's one of the first casualties of a patient's ego. If you're like me, it might first materialize through lowered self-esteem because "you" are now different from "them." Once you're diagnosed with cancer, you become once removed from everyone you know—

even your old self. Nudging away at your self-esteem will be the vanity angle (your symptoms and treatment side-effects push vanity out the window), and the acceptance angle (you may require more attention or be overly sensitive to your environment but don't want to complain and cause a fuss).

Understanding that your own comfort and peace of mind should take top priority over how others feel may seem selfish on its face but you might soon discover, as I did, that speaking your mind (tactfully but honestly) and being yourself (comfortable and without adornments) is extremely liberating. Taking this approach will actually boost your self-esteem and also the respect and understanding from those around you. Have faith that your inner circle, and even your medical team, will appreciate your honest perspective. They'll want you to be comfortable and in good spirits so you can get better faster.

It didn't take long for me to realize that no one was scrutinizing my recovery process or me. It was my own fear of attracting unwanted sympathy (pity, really) through conversations about diagnosis, prognosis and treatment. When I was in public situations, I wanted to present myself in a way that seemed reasonably together, one that insinuated everything was fine and there was no need to have a conversation about cancer. I found myself averting the gaze of others and trying to disguise any deficits. This was the beginning of me trying to shrink into myself, as if I was unworthy of attention. I was deeply self-conscious.

* * * * * * * * *

The serious nature of my tumor, and all the sudden physical impairments I was experiencing, caused my first surgery to come up very fast. This needle biopsy was crucial, not necessarily dangerous, and didn't cause too many additional side effects. But being whisked into the hospital only to fight through monumental physical therapy to regain whatever motor functions the tumor hadn't already destroyed, made it very difficult for me to be the same person I was just a few weeks earlier. It took me a while to get over my hang up of looking ill and weak. This was partly due to the fact that I was trying to grasp the rapid turn of events myself. I was still reeling over the loss of my functionality and independence.

Looking back, I realize how strong my defense mechanisms became. I was trying hard to give an appearance of progress and healing. I'd try to coordinate my movements in such a way as to insinuate everything was just fine. Giving in to my limp or asking for a hand would only subject me to the sympathies and questions of bystanders. After several months of that charade, I realized it didn't matter if my reality was exposed. No one expected me to be the same, knowing I had a tumor in my brain. I finally began to relax and carry on in my new reality, realizing everyone else already had. It was okay to be myself. Besides, pretending was exhausting. This internal conflict taught me the only thing that mattered was my own personal commitment to healing. It now allowed me to wisely avoid anything that might hinder that, including individuals who pushed my buttons, whether deliberately or not.

* * * * * * * * *

One tangent of this empowerment was realizing I was no longer concerned with the opinions of others. That doesn't mean I lost respect for their opinions, or didn't care what they thought; it's just that I no longer allowed myself to be influenced by them, to be so quick to change my position or plans merely based on someone else's differing opinion. Holding my ground was my new approach. If I felt strongly about something, it stuck. I've gained a lot more self-respect since the early days of my cancer journey. I've also gained a keener awareness of when I'm being taken advantage of, whereas in the past I was too accommodating and often felt used. Cancer opened my eyes to these personal shortfalls. Once you get to this point in your level of self-confidence, others will sense it. You'll be a force to be reckoned with. And you deserve that kind of respect.

One way to know that you've reached the pinnacle of self-confidence is when you feel a sense of calm in the midst of other people's anxieties or negativities. With a focus keenly aimed at my personal agenda of wellness and a positive attitude, I found immunity from the stress around me. Whether it was speed racers on the highway, tailgating to get me out of their way, or just a negative rant from someone around me, I was unaffected. It feels like I'm armed with an insulated force field, a stable wall of calm that protects me from any erosion of peace.

I'm fond of the new, strong and confident me. I treat others with respect and I consider myself a good role model for our kids. It's good for them to see how the stress of others fails to impact me like it once did. My personal growth, especially under such harsh conditions as cancer survival, made a big impact on my children. If I can do it, they can aspire to it.

It's never too early to teach kids that a stressed-out lifestyle is toxic. My example teaches them how to respond to stressors. With the possibility of having less time in the future for me to prepare my children for this aspect of life, I'm very mindful to use the time I have more meaningfully. As long as I'm alive, I'm one half of a parenting partnership, so far, so good. Our kids see a calm and reasonably patient Mom, available to them anytime. Finding the stronger version of yourself, for your children's sake, is one of the silver linings of cancer, there if you strive to find it. Through great difficulty, personal growth may soar by leaps and bounds.

* * * * * * * * *

On a lighter note, my self-esteem became so strong I decided to make use of all the good stuff I had acquired throughout my life. What better time to break out the good china, the expensive crystal, the guest towels? Light all the beautiful candles and wear my good jewelry? Grab the pretty handbag and wear those matching shoes (if only I could). Does this go against my earlier advice to refrain from vanity? Not really. In this case, you may choose to be whomever you feel like on a particular day. And pampering yourself is a type of reward, a way to elevate yourself to VIP status in your own life. When I was able to enjoy my good things, it was like another layer of self-esteem wrapped around my shoulders. It's a wonderful feeling when you put yourself at the head of the line. By bringing out the best in yourself and in your household, you may find, as I did, your family's spirits lifted by your own. No one loses here.

On a practical note, I will admit that I stopped accumulating stuff. Once I could see all the good stuff I already had, I realized it was quite enough for a lifetime's worth of enjoyment. Don't get me wrong, I still think it's nice to collect and value special things, I just knew I was done collecting. For example, since our first year of marriage, Rich and I have been collecting and using Spode Christmas-themed dinnerware. I'm pretty sure the set is now complete. I'll let you know if I can resist adding to our collection the next time I see an irresistibly priced addition. After eighteen years of use, we haven't broken one piece. Maybe I'll buy a replacement piece if that record run is broken.

With regard to the darker side of my scenario, I guess I didn't want to leave too long a trail for my survivors—or my replacement. Too much stuff could sadden the people who love me. It would also make for a lot of work, sorting through my lifelong accumulation of treasures once I'm gone. Every sticky note or cotton swab will emit sadness, every voicemail, tissue in the pocket, unfinished drink in the fridge, will be tinged with sorrow. At least my clothes, jewelry and Spode would definitely go to my daughter Angela. That would be simple enough. But, no, I wouldn't add to this material legacy.

* * * * * * * * *

Is it a coincidence that my choice to stop accumulating comes at a time when I'm keenly aware of my own mortality? No, how can I not be reminded of the worst-case scenario, which is also connected to how my mom died? The sadness of how we lost her is one I would never want to repeat for my own kids. Mom had been hard on her body for many years. The onset of breast cancer led to chemo and radiation, followed by a retinue of prescription drugs and alcohol abuse. She rarely left the house. Her diet was poor and she spent most of her time on the couch, mindlessly numbed by the television droning on well past the time she conked out.

I was in grad school, about forty-five minutes from home, while my mom was declining. But my regular trips back home were enough for me to be a witness to the tragedy of her last days. It was an awful existence. My heart broke for the woman I called "Mommy" until junior high. I missed the vibrant person she had been when I was younger. As much as my siblings, along with my dad, tried to pull her up and out of this purposeless existence, she proved stubborn and dug deeper into her personal hell. After our concerted efforts would be met with constant resistance, we would give up and go back to our respective businesses, schools, work, gym, friends and what not. Every so often, I remember Mom practically leaping off the couch to scold us for going out and leaving her. In retrospect, it seemed as though she was hallucinating. It pained us all that her perspective was full of resentment and without any regard to what was best for her life, or for her family's sake.

To make a long story short, she alienated her children and her husband. It was all we could do just to get her to attend my little brother's wedding. Even though she made it, while there, she was confused and uncomfortable. I was embarrassed for her. Writing this is difficult but it's hard not to think about how my own mother dealt with cancer, and how she made life so miserable for everyone around her in spite of her remission. I don't want to repeat that. Her death left a scar on me because she deteriorated mentally and physically—well beyond her cancer because much of it was self-inflicted. I don't want my own death, whenever it may occur, to be a scar on my children or my husband. I'd rather die admirably, with peace and a belief that we may all one day be united in a far better world than what we know on Earth.

The last memory I have of my mother is having to sort through all her things after she died; it fell on me, my dad, and my siblings to figure out what to do with all that she'd accumulated over the years. There was so much waste. She had clothes in the closet with tags still on them and a ridiculous amount of toiletries that merely collected dust. Her excessive shopping was probably a way to compensate for a need or emptiness in her life, most of it simply in her mind.

I don't have emptiness in my life. That's why I'm motivated to continue my personal growth. I'd rather leave a legacy of hope for my kids than memories of pain and shallow angst:

Just as a first impression is important for strangers, I believe the last impression is important for the children you leave behind.

CHAPTER 16

MEDITATION AND MASSAGE

Meditation: A way to train the mind to get into a deeper state of awareness; the act of meditating; contemplation, reflection, spiritual introspection. Learning how to meditate can teach us how to be still and let go of negativity, even if it's only for a few minutes at a time. To those who have never tried it, this may sound like an impossible achievement, especially when suffering from cancer. In my situation, meditation was a welcome escape. Focusing on breathing, the sounds of nature around me, imagining an oasis of tranquility—anything but the tumor growing inside my brain—was like an out-of-body experience that gave my psyche a break from reality. Not only was it a much-needed moment of calm during my hectic treatment days, it was also a way to cling to some semblance of sanity, to not allow my cancer to push me over the edge with incessant worry. Without meditation, I would have sunk into despair.

It's hard to understand meditation without experiencing it for yourself. You need to begin with an open mind and a positive attitude, ready to test the benefits of mental control. With practice, the process can become automatic. Once you get the hang of mental control, and decide what sensors you'll accept and which you'll reject, the physical calm will be inevitable and indescribable.

Before my diagnosis and the physical shortfalls that followed it, the concept of meditation was completely incompatible with my busy lifestyle and hyper personality. While struggling with the emotional wreck I was becoming after my diagnosis, I decided to read up on meditation, thoroughly enough to have a shot at some success. After a little digging, I came across some easy-to-understand explanations and I dove right in. One book I highly recommend is *You Can Conquer Cancer*, by Ian Gawler (new edition by Tarcher, February 2015). The chapter on meditation is easy to understand and I was surprised by how quickly I picked up the concept.

Whenever I was ready to meditate, I would choose a tranquil location, free from distractions. I'd already compiled some soothing music, in case the sounds of nature weren't going to cut it, depending on my mood. Normally, I was content with the noises of the desert and our backyard birds, water fountains, or palm tree leaves rustling in the wind. A comfortable place to sit is really important, but it's best to not get too comfortable—you don't want to fall asleep, just slip into another state of consciousness.

It's important to remember to turn off the phone and tell others you don't want to be disturbed while you take a meditation break. If you start off with five to ten minutes in the beginning and increase the time by a couple of minutes each day, you might find, as I did, the perfect allotment that offers you enough rejuvenation without being forced. One helpful hint is to try to choose a regular time of day for meditation, such as first thing in the morning or when you get home after treatments. Getting into a routine will help your mind and body fall into the habit of slowing down instead of fighting you. I looked forward to these moments and still do.

There are different types of meditation: breathing, guided, and concentration, to name a few. Each practice emphasizes its own goal. Meditation is part of several religious practices and psychophysical disciplines. You'll need to decide which is right for you.

This is how I put into practice what I had read:

With ideal weather where we live in Arizona, my meditation almost always takes place in the backyard. I like to have a blanket and sunglasses with me. I had read that you should keep your eyes open when meditating. After being seated, I align my arms and legs so that they're symmetrical. I like my hands loosely clasped, elbows resting by my hips. I ensure that both legs are doing the same thing. Once lined up, I begin concentrating on clearing my mind of thoughts. I concentrate on my body parts, starting with the feet and working my way up. During this process, I think about tensing up each muscle group, squeezing and releasing. As counter-productive as this might seem, the muscle tightening followed by releasing results in deep physical relaxation. My breathing becomes deeper and my mind clears.

As foreign as it may be for you, I suggest trying it a handful of times. You don't have to be alone and silence isn't required. Some level of meditation can be achieved as a passenger in a car, or while seated in a waiting room. Try checking your blood pressure before and after your sessions. Set your goals for length and frequency of sessions and re-evaluate after a week.

* * * * * * * * *

Oncology Massage: The modification of massage therapy techniques in order to safely work around complications of cancer and its treatment.
I was fortunate to have a friend who not only gives an incredible massage, she was also training to do oncology massage and offered to practice on me. During her training, Magda gained an understanding of the disease itself and the many ways it can affect the body, the side effects of treatment, and how to modify massage techniques in order to adapt to the side effects.

If anyone tells you it's simply an expensive treat, I would say massage is very soothing and helpful for a cancer patient. I have an oncology massage about once a month to increase blood circulation, work out stiffness, help reduce pain and fatigue. It also greatly lifts my mood. Magda, my massage therapist, usually has some sort of aromatherapy in the room, along with meditative music or nature sounds. It's a very pleasant experience that I look forward to.

I highly recommend finding a massage therapist that you feel comfortable with since you'll be spending some time with him or her naked. Expect to be very thirsty afterwards, you might have a runny nose, and you'll most definitely feel the urge to urinate. You may also feel a strong desire to sleep. If you're not feeling particularly strong, it may be best to have somebody take you to and from your appointment. Also, it doesn't hurt to check if your insurance will cover it. Before booking an appointment, make sure the massage therapist has been trained in oncology massage.

Before your treatment with an oncology massage therapist, you may be asked a series of questions. Here's a sample of what those standard intake questions touched on, in my experience:

- Cancer treatment history
- Tumor site or metastasis
- Compromised blood cell counts
- Lymph node involvement
- Blood clots or blood clot risk
- Medications (short and long term)
- Vital organ involvement
- Fragile or unstable tissue
- Medical devices
- Fatigue, neuropathy, or pain
- Changes in sensation
- Recent effects of treatment

CHAPTER 17

"WHAT, ME WORRY?"

Of all the new concepts we patients need to embrace, getting a grip on worry (and learning how not to) is probably the toughest to master but the one that gives us the most peace. But it doesn't seem possible, especially given all we have to worry about when we're facing terminal cancer. Alfred E. Newman, the *Mad Magazine* "personality," was famous for his simple quote, "What, me worry?" As a kid, I was a fan and collector of the offbeat and often-raunchy publication. I never thought much about Alfred's saying when I was younger, but now I realize he was ahead of his time. Worry is a shackle. And if I can learn how to circumvent worry while facing terminal brain cancer, then you most certainly can too. Once you do, you'll never go back to your old stressful ways again. You see, it's just that liberating.

"A man is what he thinks about all day long."
Ralph Waldo Emerson

For the religious and spiritually minded that have become familiar with (or exposed to) the Bible, you've probably read or heard about worry actually being a sin. Say what? Everbody worries. How can you be alive and not worry sometime? From the time we're born, our parents worry about our sleeping, eating, and pooping patterns and schedules. They worry about how we'll do our first time on the school bus. They worry about money, safety, politics and pollution. We grow up emulating our parents and continue the pattern of worrying.

Conversations frequently begin with, "I'm so worried about…" and "I'm worried that…" And much of the time, the worry is for nothing. Because, guess what? Worrying accomplishes absolutely nothing. Our mental energy is more productively used in positive thinking and positive conversation. I'm not saying that worry has no place whatsoever. We wouldn't be human without concerns, feeling the need to protect and do what needs to be done for self-preservation. Constructive worry or rumination can help us find solutions by weighing out the pros and cons of a problem. I have found myself able to put a concern aside temporarily, and let my dream state work on it. Many mornings, I'd wake up with an idea and the energy to solve the problem that weighed on my mind the night before.

Worrying is as natural as eating and breathing. It's ever-present and constant, in thought and in speech. But it doesn't have to be. Think about that possibility. Whether you have spiritual beliefs or not, you can make the switch from non-productive worry to deliberate, proactive response to whatever stressor crosses your path. This is what happened with me and by no means did this process take place overnight. I wasn't enjoying the tightness in my chest and the tension across my shoulders. After recognizing the physical affects of stress, such as noticing my breathing wasn't right, I began paying attention to the patterns of what stressed me out. I also learned ways to diminish worry with mental exercises and changing my stream of consciousness. One of the first things I did was take notice of the source of my stress. Was it my condition, a weakness or impediment, a person, a test result? Then I try to deliberately shift my mental focus away from whatever that stressor is, for as long as I can and hope that decreases its impact on my anxiety. If possible, I'll move away from any distractions and try to give my mind a rest. It's so important to be kind to yourself and take a break now and then. Trust me, your mind can get used to rest periods.

When you find something that alleviates worry and stress, go back to it. For me, it was walking my dog, petting my cats, reading a magazine (unrelated to health), calling or texting a friend, getting on Facebook. Interacting with my pets or my friends started out as distractions but ended up being therapeutic. Also, don't underestimate the power of nature. Go outside and try to enjoy a park or your own backyard. Nature is a major comfort for me, the greatest supplier of sweet and attractive sights, smells and sounds.

As much as I enjoy reading books and articles about healing cancer, I realized one day during that first summer of treatments that I needed a fiction book. My neighbor Tina had passed on a book that provided just the diversion I needed, called *The Perfect Summer*, by Luanne Rice (Bantam, 2003), and it took place in a small New England town on the coast. This connection to my native East Coast roots gave me a lot of comfort with its descriptions of familiar scenery and likable characters. I almost gave that book away before giving it a chance, telling myself there was no time for fun or fiction. Maybe, but it had a place. The next summer, I found another work of fiction (different author, similar location) and I tore through it enthusiastically when the mood struck.

Even more important to me than fiction, however, is the Bible. I refer to this passage often. It's from Matthew 6:25-34. I'd like to share it with you:

Therefore I say to you, do not worry about your life, what you will eat or what you will drink; not about your body, what you will put on. Is not life more than food and the body more than clothing? Look at the birds of the air, for they neither sow nor reap nor gather into barns, yet your heavenly Father feeds them. Are you not of more value than they? Which of you by worrying can add one cubit to his stature?

So why do you worry about clothing? Consider the lilies of the field, how they grow: they neither toil nor spin; and yet I say to you that even Solomon in all his glory was not arrayed like one of these. Now if God so clothes the grass of the field, which today is, and tomorrow is thrown into the oven, will He not much more clothe you, O you of little faith?

Therefore do not worry, saying, "What shall we eat?" or "What shall we drink?" or "What shall we wear?" For after all these things the Gentiles seek. For your heavenly Father knows that you need all these things. But seek first the kingdom of God and His righteousness, and all these things shall be added to you. Therefore do not worry about tomorrow, for tomorrow will worry about its own things. Sufficient for the day is its own trouble.

CHAPTER 18

POST-OP RECOVERY AND HOME SAFETY

One of the most important cancer transitions you need to prepare for is learning your own physical limitations. Once symptoms take over and treatments begin, you'll be more vulnerable to all kinds of accidents due to an inability to negotiate what used to be normal tasks and obstacles. Surgery, in particular, will require you to get on the fast track of making your surroundings safe enough for post-op recovery. Brain cancer patients will be especially prone to mobility issues, very frustrating and potentially very dangerous.

The nice people at the hospital told us about patient-proofing the house. Here is a list of what we did to make my recovery at home as safe as possible.

Move area rugs and make a clear path in the rooms you frequent: I had to use a walker after my needle biopsy (Round One, my first surgery) and the leg of the walker got caught on a corner of the area rug. Falling in a room full of furniture is very dangerous.

Get a shower seat: Treatments can wear you out. Take a break in the shower and be safe at the same time by sitting. It will also give peace of mind to your caregivers. Our shower had a built-in seat, which turned out to be a necessity.

Install shower bars and handles in the shower or other areas of the bathroom: Better safe than sorry and they really are convenient, even when you're fully recovered. I didn't need a shower bar during Round One but I needed one after the craniotomy (Round 2, tumor removal). Even if you doubt you'll need a safety rail in the shower, have one installed anyway. There's no benefit to testing your balancing act.

Get a bath mat with a thick, rubber, nonskid backing: We found ours at Home Goods. If your shower has no grab bars to help you exit onto the mat, I suggest installing a couple just in case.

Install a hand-held shower sprayer: You can always swap it out when you no longer need it. But they're also helpful in cleaning the shower walls, so you may decide to keep it.

Camp downstairs if your house isn't single story and your bedroom is upstairs: You'll need to get the green light from your physical therapist to negotiate stairs. Plan on not going upstairs for a while.

Install a railing along the staircase if you don't already have a banister: The possibility of losing your balance while negotiating stairs makes it absolutely necessary to have a railing to grab hold of. Also, going up is a lot easier than going down.

* * * * * * * * *

Just because you're on a treatment plan of chemotherapy and/or radiation, doesn't mean over-the-counter meds won't be recommended. While some are helpful, many aren't really necessary. My advice is to listen to your body before simply taking pills as ordered. You might find you don't need them, after all.

While in the hospital recovering from my first surgery, the needle biopsy, I was told I would be taking Prilosec. This was explained as a necessity. I assumed it was for heartburn but they explained it was for preventing acid due to stress. I didn't really get the connection but I was exhausted and feeling like I wasn't in charge, so I just took it. The nurses also insisted on taking Tylenol on a regular basis. But since I didn't have headaches, I didn't take them. A stool softener was also recommended, but I opted to take care of that problem with food and good nutrition.

Get to know your body and listen to your instincts. You don't have to take all of the over-the-counter meds that are suggested. Nature can take care of many of the body's processes. If you need a couple Tums® or Tylenol® capsules, you'll know. But try to abstain from the regular ingestion of drugs you really don't need.

CHAPTER 19

PHYSICAL THERAPY

One of the toughest aspects of brain cancer is negotiating the stroke-like symptoms associated with tumor growth. As if dealing with the side effects of radiation and chemo weren't enough, add to the list trying to regain your mobility, balance, and speech. Physical therapy is a must. But it's not easy, especially because you'll be tired from the traditional treatment plan of being zapped and injected with toxic chemicals.

To motivate myself to push through regular physical therapy, I would think *Re-Train the Brain* while doing repetitive exercises, and *Repave the Brainwaves* while trying to persuade muscle memory to kick back in. It was encouraging to know that the brain really does have something like muscle memory. I was determined to give my brain and body a loud wake up call.

I desperately wanted to be back at my previous level of activity but small accomplishments would have to suffice at this stage in my recovery. The first surgery (needle biopsy) didn't have as many challenges as the craniotomy (tumor removal). Having been down this road twice, it's my expert opinion that repeated activities of daily living (occupational therapists refer to them as ADLs), helped me to progress more quickly than the prescribed exercises. However, all therapies helped me, and I recommend participating in any and all that are recommended for you; it's well worth the time and effort.

Here are some of my favorite physical activities:

- Small movements with light weights or stretchy bands
- Lots of stretching
- Yoga
- Swimming (my favorite, no strain, water gives adequate resistance for building strength, and it feels great)

During physical therapy, repeat to yourself, or say out loud, encouraging words or phrases while performing your program, or during unstructured activity. The repetitive nature of this act can reinforce what you're doing via the mind-body connection. Physical therapy can be boring at times and it's not always pain free. Music you love will also help motivate you through these tough moments.

Squeezing in special, rehabilitative exercises throughout my entire day became somewhat of a game for me, so badly did I want to increase my strength and comfort. For example, while I waited for the blender to finish my smoothie, I would do push-ups standing up against the counter or wall. While I folded clothes, seated on the floor, I would do a lot of stretching. While standing in line at the check out counter, I would do hip or neck rotations, or stretch my triceps. The bottom line to physical therapy is to keep it continuous and seize the opportunity to advance your progress with creativity. That's how you can fast-forward your strength, flexibility and, ultimately, your recovery. The power is in your hands.

The physical therapy exercises given to me were broken up into upper body, lower body, fine motor, core, and stretching. Your therapist will design a program that's just right for you and your needs.

Here's a general list of what I did:

Lower body: My sessions began with 15 minutes on a stationary bike. At home, before leaving the house, I walked the dog, did some deep breathing and hydrated.

Lower body exercises (get details from your PT): Bridging; quadruples; sit-to-stand; thigh push; flex foot against resistance band; side leg kicks; toe taps; weight shifting; leg kicks to the front, sides and back; marching in place with knees high while maintaining balance; step-down/step-up; mini squat; side step with tubing; side-step with squat; leg extensions using tubing.

Examples of Upper body exercises: Tricep extensions; wall ball circles; wood chops; up and outs with ball; towel slide on wall; bicep curls with dumbbells or stretchy band; push-ups.

Stretching (I found it helpful to watch myself in the mirror because my left arm would get lazy and it helped to "talk" to it): Use a stretchy band to stretch weaker calf; stretch arms overhead and in front of chest; stretch legs standing and spread out on floor; holding each position for 10-15 seconds in each direction.

Core Exercises (improves your balance and stability by training the muscles in the pelvis, lower back, hips and abdomen to work in harmony): bridges; planks; crunches; leg lifts while lying on your back, raising legs and holding just a few inches above the floor.

Fine Motor Exercises (for stroke-like symptoms): Using your weak hand, stack and un-stack coins; purchase therapeutic putty and pinch, pull and squeeze it; fold laundry; use a dry erase board and marker to practice writing; practice typing; gripper squeezes; stress ball squeezes;

open mail; tap fingers; touch each finger to thumb, and try to build up speed; do palm flips (turn weaker hand over as quickly as you can).

I found it helpful to think deliberately about any action I was performing with my left hand since that was my weak side. If I lost my focus, objects would just drop to the floor. I would say to myself, "I am now carrying this bottle of wine. Maintain the grip!" Usually works like a charm. I controlled things better by squeezing onto the object and reminding myself of the task at hand.

I gained back a lot of fine motor and cognitive skills by planning meals and following through with the steps from start to finish. I'd choose a recipe, shop for ingredients, and gather all the utensils (measuring cups, etc). Unscrewing caps and lids is a good exercise for an underused hand. Some recipes required math and a steady hand. Cutting and peeling successfully (without injuries) built my confidence. I valued being able to help with meals. If and when fatigue set in, I would sit during the prep part.

CHAPTER 20

TRAVELING WITH CANCER

Throughout the past two-and-a-half years, I've experienced various levels of independence and dependence. At my worst, I found mobility with a walker, a cane, holding onto someone's arm, and scaling furniture. At the time of this writing, I was walking but not feeling confident in my balance. I had a couple of minor falls, minor because I didn't completely collapse and land on the floor or the ground. Each incident had to do with me making a mistake in hand placement on whatever I was gripping, or a lack of coordination with the rest of my body. Even without injuries, it's very disturbing to lose control of one's body.

As I was going through my second round of chemo and radiation, our family went on vacation for three weeks; two in Massachusetts with the kids and family, and one week just me and Rich, at the Real Resort in Playa Del Carmen, Mexico. I desperately wanted to be pain free and get around more swiftly. But throughout the vacation, I didn't take any risks. I relied on others to hold my hand while going about. Rich and I found all the short cuts around the resort to save me steps. When possible, I'd park myself at some comfortable, scenic spot while Rich fetched our pool towels and drinks. We were always looking for ways to preserve my energy.

Yes, there were a few times when both of us got frustrated due to my deficits and difficulties. But, overall, it was an incredible week, full of laughs, sun, and delicious food. I stuck to my strict ketogenic diet, except for a couple of meals at this special place called *Chef's Plate*. The staff at the resort made it clear they would provide for special dietary needs. All we had to do was ask. "Don't hesitate, you deserve it," they said. So, I vowed to get right back on my diet. Don't be afraid to ask for customized meals or aids in your mobility. Most resorts and hotels are more than willing to accommodate their guests. If traveling meant you would have to take health risks, you might be reluctant to venture out. It would be a shame to limit the experiences you can share with your loved ones. It doesn't have to be that way. It just takes planning, perseverance, and common sense.

Tip: Regarding footwear: For those with weakness on one side and/or foot drop, it can be difficult to find shoes you can get around in safely and comfortably. But my experience is that practical shoes don't work for dressy occasions. If you've got an event to attend, start looking for smart shoes ahead of time, and give those shoes a dress rehearsal.

While we were at the resort in Mexico, I mostly got around barefoot since we were outside the majority of the time. But I also brought along a neutral pair of Skechers for all-purpose use. My left-side weakness, caused by brain or nerve damage, caused me to have a limp and frequent toe stubbing. It can also be painful walking distances. Skechers slip-ons were the solution for me, and they were reasonably priced. Flip-flops are a staple here in blistering-hot Arizona, but they're not the safest choice in my situation. Crocs™ brand is my pick if you have trouble keeping shoes on your feet and you require comfort.

CHAPTER 21

A JOB FOR SUPERMAN

It was between Thanksgiving and Christmas of 2013 that we realized things were changing; my progress was reversing. Just like the very first symptoms, these were gradual. My left leg was weakening and some of my fine motor skills were getting worse. Having been down this road before, I had a sense of peace that there might be some hope, something to hold onto, and that I didn't need to break down and lose control. Perhaps it was this little thing called faith. Of course, there was worry and fear of the unknown, as well.

After a year of treatments and the strict ketogenic diet (used as an adjuvant therapy to minimize tumor growth), I felt like I was getting back to normal. I started giving in to sugary foods beginning with one slice of birthday cake in July, which led to other sweets and starches throughout the rest of that year. I've since realized, you've got to keep supportive people around you that will slap your hand and help keep you on track.

In November, my MRI showed a small spot but I didn't feel a recurrence of symptoms so I didn't worry too much about it. But a month later, the next MRI showed an additional growth, in the same area. At the same time, I started to regain my limp, a loss of grip in my left hand, and short-term memory loss; that Michigan accent was also making a come back. My professional team decided to draw blood for tests; chemotherapy would resume.

* * * * * * * * *

If you're newly diagnosed, you may not yet know if surgery is an option, when the impossible suddenly becomes a possibility. I had seen many posts on brain tumor support pages about second, third, and even fifth tumor removals and craniotomies. But I didn't for one moment think I would be a candidate after being told in early 2012 that my tumor was inoperable. Sure, I thought once or twice about whether there might be some superhuman neurosurgeon who might possess the skill and technique for reaching in and safely removing this puppy. Rich and I already had our team in place and these supermen and superwomen could see the tumor was too deep in my thalamus for safe removal. Radiation and chemo was the only option at the time.

Make no mistake, Rich and I did daily research, aggressively keeping up on the latest news and techniques in the neuro world. We reached out and networked all we could. But when my MRIs came back in late 2013 showing change/growth, and the Temodar wasn't doing anything, we started to get nervous. That's when I reached out to my brain cancer buddy Melissa, who had been traveling down this road for a year longer than I had. I didn't expect her to have an immediate idea or answer to our fear of a dead end in treatment. But, to my surprise, she had a number and a name, and the green light to contact her Dr. Superman.

We sent an email and soon Rich was in deep discussion with Melissa's surgeon, Dr. Nader Sanai, the partner and colleague of Dr. Kris Smith, the surgeon who performed my needle biopsy in March 2012. This was an unbelievable coincidence.

****

Dr. Sanai accessed my MRIs and medical records. Here are relevant excerpts from his notes, following an office visit after his review of my medical history:

Dictated on: March 5, 2014

OFFICE NOTE

Diagnosis: MALIGNANT NEOPLASM OF FRONTAL LOBE OF BRAIN

Event Chronology
03/09/2012 Right needle biopsy, enhancing thalamic lesion, anaplastic astrocytoma, Kris Smith, M.D.

History of Present Illness
History From: Patient
Chief Complaint: Brain Tumor
Referring MD: Donald J. Lauer, MD
Visit Type: Follow-up Visit

This is a 46-year-old female with a history of a right enhancing thalamic lesion for which she underwent stereotactic needle biopsy on March 9, 2012. At the time, final pathology returned anaplastic astrocytoma, MIB-1=8.9%. She completed standard radiation therapy with temozolomide, and completed one year of maintenance temozolomide. Postoperatively, she experienced continued speech difficulty, and left-sided hemiparesis which has gradually improved. Most recent MRI scan dated February 25, 2014 demonstrates interval increase in size of focus of enhancement centrally. She is here today to discuss neurosurgical intervention.

Plan

Right frontal craniotomy for tumor resection with asleep motor mapping.
T1 WAND MRI with diffusion tensor imaging.

Problems Added

Neoplasm of unspecified nature of brain

New Orders

Surgery Recommended

During that office visit, Dr. Sanai thrilled us with the declaration, "I think I can get this thing out." How mind-blowing (pardon the pun). A new option. We discussed the risks and the benefits. For me, there really wasn't any other choice but to go ahead with it. Dr. Sanai is an expert in intra-operative brain mapping, a diagnostic guide during that helps a surgeon navigate tumor removal while preserving vital functions. That was comforting info.

I remember thinking, "Let's move with this before it becomes just a fantasy." We had lots of arrangements to make between caring and supervision for the kids, and just getting me squared away and ready to do this.

There were a few things that had to be done before the day of surgery. A mapping MRI, chest X-ray, blood work and, of course, sharing this news with family and friends. I started feeling like I was getting ready to have another baby, packing my bag to leave at a moment's notice. Speaking of which, here's a list of things I brought with me to the hospital: a bathrobe; pants with a stretchy waist; lip balm; a white-noise machine; personal toiletries; button-up shirts; slipper socks; headphones; hairbands/clips.

On March 9th, my sister-in-law arrived to take care of the kids. On the 13th, my surgery took place. Dr. Sanai was able to successfully remove the entire tumor. This was a job for Superman and my own Dr. Superman came through. Believe it or not, I was able to get up out of my hospital bed the very next day, using a walker. Within a week, I was discharged from inpatient rehab and happily back at home.

Next in line was Round 2 of radiation and chemotherapy. The doctor explained we would have to treat the tumor bed and the flair, both new terms for us. What an unpleasant surprise. I was sure I was done with radiation, but now that I knew my tumor was completely removed, this was a small price to pay for peace of mind.

CHAPTER 22

DR. NADER SANAI: TUMOR RESECTION

On March 13, 2014, Dr. Nader Sanai of the Barrow Neurological Institute in Phoenix, Arizona, performed a tumor resection of my originally inoperable brain tumor, utilizing intra-operative brain mapping in order to preserve brain functionality. It was successful in that he was able to remove the entire tumor. I have no doubt that I wouldn't have been able to write this book and live this long had it not been for Dr. Sanai.

Here are some excerpts of his surgical notes, obtained from my medical records. I wanted to share them because I think they're fascinating and show the importance of what these amazing professionals can do.

Operative Report

Operation
Date of Procedure: 03/13/2014

PREOPERATIVE DIAGNOSIS: *Right frontal high-grade glioma.*
POSTOPERATIVE DIAGNOSIS: *Right frontal high-grade glioma.*

NAME OF PROCEDURE:

1. *Stealth neuronavigation.*
2. *Operating microscope.*
3. *Right frontal craniotomy for resection of tumor.*
4. *Intraoperative cortical and subcortical stimulation mapping, initial hour of physician attendance.*
5. *Intraoperative cortical and subcortical stimulation mapping, second hour of physician attendance.*
6. *Intraoperative cortical and subcortical stimulation mapping, third hour of physician attendance.*
7. *Intraoperative cortical language mapping, fourth hour of physician attendance.*
8. *Intraoperative cortical and subcortical stimulation mapping, fifth hour of physician attendance.*

SURGEON: *Nader Sanai, MD*

ANESTHESIA: *General*

DESCRIPTION OF PROCEDURE: *The patient was brought to the operating room, underwent general endotracheal intubation. Appropriate lines and monitors were placed. The patient was placed supine on the operating table, the head was placed into 3-point fixation in the Mayfield device. Preoperatively obtained volumetric MRI imaging was transferred to the Stealth Medtronic neuronavigational system and registered to the patient's cranium. Accuracy was confirmed, and a linear incision overlying the right frontal lobe was marked, prepped, and draped in the usual fashion.*

An incision made sharply with a 10 blade. Bipolar electrocautery was used for hemostasis. Rany clips were applied and the scalp flap was retracted with scalp hooks. The round-cutting Anspach drill was used to place a bur hole inferiorly, and the side-cutter was used to turn a craniotomy overlying the right frontal lobe. The bone flap was elevated with a Penfield 3. Peripheral tack-up sutures were placed with 4-0 nylon stitches. The operating microscope was draped and brought into the field.

Using standard microdissection techniques, the dura was opened with a 15 blade and a dural guide, and the leaflets were held in place with 4-0 Nurolon stitches. At this point, the intraoperative cortical subcortical stimulation mapping protocol was initiated using an Ojemann stimulator at 60 Hz frequency, 1 msec pulse duration, with 5-7 mA per channel. The cortical motor threshold for arm motor function was 6.7 mA per channel. This was used to identify the motor cortex. A trajectory to the tumor anterior to the motor cortex by 2 gyri was then undertaken using a combination of bipolar electrocautery, microscissors, and standard microdisection techniques. This subcortical trajectory of the tumor then enabled additional subcortical motor mapping at thresholds much lower ranging from 2-5 mg per channel. This subcortical tumor motor mapping enabled us to completely resect the tumor in its entirety, taking care to preserve the integrity of the descending cortical spinal tracts.

Once tumor resection was completed, the area was copiously irrigated and inspected. The dura was closed with 4-0 Nurolon stitches in watertight fashion. The bone flap was reapproximated with a titanium plating system. The galea was closed with interrupted 3-0 Vicryl stitches. The skin was closed with 4-0 monofilament.

The patient was moved out of pin fixation and extubated.

ESTIMATED BLOOD LOSS: 100 cc.

SPECIMEN SENT: Labeled brain tumor.

* * * * * * * * *

The following is a pathology report of the tumor that was removed from my brain, obtained from my medical records and dated March 13, 2014, the day of my surgery:

Neuropathology Report

Clinical Information: *Right brain tumor*

Specimen Submitted: *Right brain tumor*

Gross Description
Received fresh are multiple fragments of tan-pink soft tissue aggregating to 0.2 x 0.2 x 0.1 cm. A smear preparation is performed and the specimen is entirely frozen on one chuck.

Frozen Section diagnosis: *Consistent with recurrent glioma*

The remainder of the previously frozen soft tissue is subsequently submitted for permanent section.

Microscopic Description
1. Sections of brain demonstrate a hypercellular astrocytoma with high grade malignant features. Neoplastic cells are large, atypical, and haphazardly arranged. Necrosis and mitotic figures are not identified. Normal-appearing brain is not identified.

Diagnosis
1. Right brain tumor, biopsy:
 - Consistent with recurrent high-grade glioma, pending review of additional material.

ADDENDA

Addendum Diagnosis:
1-2. Right brain tumor, biopsy and permanent:
Consistent with recurrent high-grade glioma.

* * * * * * * * * *

The following is an excerpt from Dr. Sanai's post-surgical report, dated March 26, 2014:

Diagnosis:
Neoplasm of unspecified nature of brain.
Malignant neoplasm of frontal lobe of brain.

Event Chronology
03/09/2012 Right needle biopsy, enhancing thalamic lesion, anaplastic astrocytoma, Kris Smith, MD.
03/13/2014 Right frontal craniotomy for resection of tumor with asleep motor mapping.

History of Present Illness
History From: Patient
Chief Complaint: Status post brain tumor
Referring MD: Donald J. Lauer, MD
Visit Type: Postoperative visit #1

This is a 46-year-old female post right frontal craniotomy for resection of previously biopsied anaplastic astrocytoma. Final pathology was consistent with recurrent anaplastic astrocytoma. She reports that she is getting better each day. Left upper extremity weakness is improving in strength and control. She is able to ambulate with a cane, and able to function at home with minimal assistance. She reports mild headaches, which are relieved with Tylenol. She denies nausea, vomiting, or seizures. Incision is clean, dry and intact. She is accompanied by her husband and father, and remains in good spirits.

CHAPTER 23

ZAP THE FLAIR, I DON'T CARE

After finishing thirty-three radiation sessions in 2012, I didn't think I would ever see the inside of the "vault" again. Rich and I believed I had received a lifetime's maximum. But return I did. The goal for this round was to specifically target any hidden cells that might be lurking around the tumor bed, getting ready to rear their ugly heads at any time and become aggressive.

The diagnostic findings after Dr. Sanai removed my tumor included a recommendation for additional radiation and chemotherapy. Here's an excerpt from my medical records dated March 26, 2014:

Radiographic/Diagnostic Findings
Gross total resection on postop MRI.

Assessment/Plan
Assessment
The patient is a 46-year-old female post right frontal craniotomy for resection of anaplastic astrocytoma. The left-sided hemiparesis is improving. She is doing well and gradually returning to her neurological baseline.

Plan

1. *Recommended follow up with Dr. McBride to consider possible role of re-irradiation.*
2. *Continued follow up with Dr. Shapiro for ongoing chemotherapy recommendations.*
3. *Molecular profiling results are pending.*
4. *Two-week Decadron taper.*
5. *Follow up with next interval MRI.*

* * * * * * * * *

We saw some of the same radiation staff that attended to me in Round One. I was pleased that I recalled some of their names. With twelve new sessions on the calendar, I had my treatment planning MRI and other types of tests in order to get ready. A new mask was designed for me and, before I knew it, I was back in position in the vault, locked into place, inhaling that familiar metallic smell that swirled in and out of the ventilated mask. I started to pray—my list was longer, too many people fighting too many battles.

Now that we exhausted every traditional treatment option (I guess chemo could go on for as long as I could stand it), and had the tumor successfully removed, the ketogenic diet became even more important to me. By now, it had become a way of life. But even so, Rich and I made even more of a concentrated commitment to the diet, timed to coincide with these last radiation treatments. The experts that were guiding me, from BNI and St. Joseph's (whose contributions to this book you'll read in Part II), informed us early on that the KD was believed to be effective when used in conjunction with radiation. That's why they call it an "adjuvant therapy." I was on full-force during Round One and felt great, the symptoms were reversing, and it's simply a very healthy way to eat. But then I fell off the wagon and the symptoms came back. I can't risk falling off the wagon this time. My options are running out.

The twelve vault visits flew right by, along with my hair.

PART II

THE KETOGENIC DIET

CHAPTER 1

WHY THE KD? WHY THE HELL NOT?

While cancer may immediately turn all your focus onto the science behind your disease and the traditional ways to treat it, the science of overall good health is also very important. It will help you progress from the harsh side effects from radiation and chemotherapy, and hopefully get you close to remission that much faster. Depending on your level of activity and general health and fitness before cancer, you may need to sign up for some personal training and pick up some reading material on your area of interest regarding fitness and nutrition. If you get admitted into the hospital early on, like I did, you may receive some in-patient physical therapy (often necessary for brain surgery recovery) and be directed to an in-patient, short-term rehabilitation program before you get the all clear to finally go home. At this point, you may as well be prepared for exercise to become a daily part of your life, if it isn't already. This will give you the best odds for regaining your strength and improving any loss of motor function.

I had a decent foundation of regular exercise and that accelerated my healing. My weight was normal and I had good muscle tone. It also helped that I already had an excellent diet. If you don't have these things, a cancer diagnosis is a great motivator, and you can fall into a positive routine very quickly. Of course, everyone is different, and the pace of progress will vary according to your abilities or your limitations. But it's never too late to adopt good habits, and the mental benefits are just as healing as the physical ones.

With cancer in my life now, the focus on nutrition was bumped up a notch. My discovery of the Ketogenic Diet (KD) in early 2012 gave me hope that fighting cancer on a metabolic level could improve my prognosis. According to the KD guidelines, I went ahead with the elimination of almost all sugar and carbs. I strongly believe this played a major role in boosting my immune system and allowing me to resume a regular exercise regimen not too long after the first surgery (the needle biopsy), and round one of radiation and chemo. I admit, there were some days when I felt that just performing my daily tasks was a workout. On those days, I tried to at least stretch my muscles.

Whether you're fighting disease or not, a "clean" diet is essential, especially for preventative care. For a cancer patient, "clean" means the Ketogenic Diet, for many biological reasons that are described in the next two chapters, by the professionals who helped me at the Barrow Neurological Institute (BNI) and St. Joseph's Hospital, both in Phoenix, Arizona.

* * * * * * * * *

We first heard about the KD through our own research, having come across articles about Otto Warburgh's research on cancer as a metabolic disease, which led to more current articles on this kind of research by Dr. Thomas Seyfried, a longtime ketogenic researcher at Boston College (and also the author of an extensive book on this subject, *Cancer as a Metabolic Disease: On the Origin, Management, and Prevention of Cancer,* John Wilcy & Sons, 2012). The KD also kept coming up in casual conversation and on Facebook among people who were using it on a regular basis. It became clear there was credibility to this method of eating. And after all, what did I have to lose? The science behind it made sense. That logic boosted my faith in it, so I decided to explore further and give it a try.

The science behind ketosis was familiar to me, from when I did the popular Atkins Diet in the late 1990s to lose weight after the birth of our first child. Unlike the Atkins, however, the ketogenic diet is not a fad. It's been used and studied since the early 1900s with plenty of success for epilepsy patients and for other brain-related issues. But I'll let the professionals discuss that in the next two chapters. One of the biggest positives about the KD is its simplicity. And, no, I don't mean to say the diet itself isn't a little complicated—at first, anyway. What I mean is, after only hearing about chemo, radiation, surgery—all these toxic or invasive methods professionals insist are the only tried and true options for treating cancer (and in the majority of cases, that may be true), it piqued my interest to learn about making my insides healthier and maybe slow the tumor growth with *good* stuff—natural foods and fats—rather than poisons, beams, scalpels, and drills.

Sure, there were new therapies and other types of meds being discussed for upcoming clinical trials, or already in clinical trials, but those wouldn't be available for years. There was really no other alternative, and no comparison in the form of food versus toxic medications. This was very appealing to me. *Bring it on and bring it on now.* I couldn't get enough information about it. I ate it all up (no kidding). I was excited and enthusiastic, full of hope. This was something I could do, and it wasn't going to be difficult with Rich at my side, taking on the KD with me.

* * * * * * * * *

The very first step in getting started was communicating to friends and family what I was about to embark on. They needed to know my KD "dos and don'ts" so they could be part of the team. I might say something like, "Please don't bring me any sweets when visiting. They're fine for the kids but very tempting for me and hard to resist." It's important for me to stick to my no-sugar policy in order to succeed with the KD. Most people understood but still, it's a tough call, cutting out sugar and carbs. These things are everywhere!

The biggest benefit I found, early on, was that the elimination of sugar, carbs, and processed foods actually took away the cravings for sugar, carbs and processed foods. This became a weapon, a tool, a tactic to stay focused and to resist off-limits stuff. We had to do some clearing out of the "contraband" within our kitchen and pantry. I threw out all the rice, pasta, and cereal. Rich and I both learned to enjoy our coffee without sweetener, and we switched from half-and-half to heavy cream (high fat, low carb). All this may sound minor but, for us, they represented breaking decades of daily practice.

Next was a trip to the grocery store. We had to shop differently and at different places. We also had to cook differently, using different types of vegetables, oils, and herbs. We started watching *The Food Network* and chatting with our friends about recipes more often, asking if anyone had an herb garden, and so forth.

We got much more familiar with the KD team at BNI, where I was being treated with traditional therapies (radiation on my brain tumor and oral chemotherapy). We went down to Dr. Adrienne Scheck's lab to have a tour and learn more about her tumor research, mainly about the metabolism of cancer cells (her contribution is in Chapter 2.) She was so happy to have somebody interested in what she had been researching for years. We also worked very closely with Lee Renda, the registered dietician nutritionist and KD expert at BNI. Lee provided me with recipes and KetoCal® supplements; she also directed me to the keto calculator website (the link is available at the end of this book in a list of handy references), a very important tool to gauge KD progress. Lee offers a lot of her expertise in Chapters 3 and 4, coming up.

* * * * * * * * *

I became acquainted with a cancer survivor on Facebook named Elaine Cantin. I read her book, *The Cantin Ketogenic Diet* (2012). I still refer to it often when I have specific questions and when I need some recipes to mix things up. Elaine has a wealth of information in her book and she welcomes questions about the KD and her experience with it on her Facebook page.

There's no doubt it's a challenging diet to follow. But if you feel you have decent willpower, and you're motivated to survive, you really owe it to yourself to give it a try. The difficulty, of course, lies in resisting sugar and carbs. Unfortunately, these are often included in every single meal and snack we come across in today's assortment of processed foods. Genetically modified organisms (GMOs), and other scientifically modified ingredients further complicate the American diet. We don't really know what's in our food so it's best to eat the purest and cleanest foods you possibly can. Since the list of low-carb foods is relatively small, I find it's not that complicated to eat this way. Also, there are books, articles and phone apps that can guide you with carb content so it's not so overwhelming to keep track of it all.

When I started the KD, we bought a food scale so we could weigh and measure our food, to the gram. My husband, Rich, followed the diet with me, which made it a lot easier to adapt it into our household. A huge challenge for us was when our friends, neighbors, and church members were preparing and delivering meals to us. Many of these dishes included ingredients we couldn't eat. They were great for the kids though. The generous efforts of all these wonderful people saved us a lot of time, money and work. We were, and continue to be, very grateful for that.

Having forbidden foods in front of us certainly presented a challenge—one that we had to overcome. There were many times they were almost too difficult to resist, like when the deliveries included mashed potatoes with butter melting on top, or some of my favorite desserts. Some of these dishes looked so scrumptious, I wrapped them up in plastic, or put them in Tupperware and stored them in the freezer for a later date. I knew at the time this was a silly idea, but I didn't care. I was feeling so deprived, this was one way I could deal with the temptation. I told myself I would continue to follow the rules, knowing there was light at the end of the tunnel.

Lee Renda, the hospital dietician told us the most important time to be on the KD was during radiation treatment. I wasn't sure at the time if we would ever find out if this was true but, with so few tools in the toolbox, I was going to do anything that held the promise of recovery. I knew the radiation treatments would last for seven weeks. I looked forward to the end of that timeframe as the possible date I could start eating normally.

With the benefit of hindsight (and isn't that the value of this book?), knowing how quickly the cancer can go from "dormant" to "aggressive-seek-and-destroy," depending on the energy supply you deny it (with the KD), or feed it (with sugars and carbs), I'd rather reprogram my eating habits than possibly face a feeding tube in my future. If you're a cancer patient, I urge you to do your best to stick with the KD. Stay strong and keep telling yourself that the long-term prospect of lengthening your life is more valuable than the short-term pleasure of eating anything you want. The inner strength you'll gain will keep building each time you resist junk food.

Brain cancer aside, it's a very healthy way to eat. I noticed my skin clear up and my nails grow long and strong. They had never done that before. Also, I was plagued with acne since the age of thirteen. Suddenly, I had none. My hair grew back curly and healthy. Everyone is different but with all these benefits, why not try the diet—without viewing it as a diet? View it as a technique that could very well lengthen your life. View it as your "new normal."

CHAPTER 2

METABOLISM OF CANCER CELLS
Adrienne C. Scheck, Ph.D.
Barrow Brain Tumor Research Center

We are living in a time of unprecedented advances in our understanding of the genetic basis of diseases, such as malignant brain tumors. Whereas the diagnosis of brain tumors has typically been done by a pathologist skilled in the diagnosis of neurological disease from the observation of tumor tissue, advances in our understanding of molecular biology have provided additional data to further define not only disease type but also to provide hints as to the prognosis and the potential for successful therapeutic intervention.

Perhaps the most important advances have been those demonstrating that tumors previously thought to be one tumor type (such as glioblastoma) might in fact have different *subtypes* due to differences in their genetic makeup. This suggests a reason why there is variability in patient prognosis, as well as the tumor's response to therapy. In fact, the analyses of genetic differences in tumors have led to the suggestion that therapies may be tailored to the particular *genetic type* of a given tumor, so-called "personalized medicine."

This is not a new goal, and quite a few therapies targeting the particular molecular characteristics of tumor cells have been tested. To date, these new therapies have met with very limited success in brain tumors. This is likely due to the fact that not all cells in a person's tumor will have any one particular therapeutic target—a phenomenon called "heterogeneity." Cells without the particular molecular traits being targeted will not be killed by that therapy.

Unlike most molecular traits, one thing found in virtually all tumor cells is *aberrant metabolism*. In the 1920s, Otto Warburg showed that tumor cells use glucose differently than normal cells.[1, 2] Tumor cells are willing to give up some of the energy they could get from glucose in order to have what they need to make more cells. For this reason, tumor cells require large amounts of glucose to ensure they have enough energy to live *and* produce more cells. If you could reduce blood glucose, you might be able to reduce tumor growth. The one caveat to this idea is that normal cells, especially those in the brain, also need glucose for energy. Thus, simply reducing glucose would harm normal tissue as well as the tumor.

One way around that would be to provide an alternate energy source for normal cells, one that cannot be used by tumor cells. *Ketones* fit this requirement, and they can be elevated in the blood by fasting, severe caloric restriction or the use of a high fat, low carbohydrate/protein diet, such as the Ketogenic Diet. The ketogenic diet has a long history of use for the treatment of pediatric epilepsy in patients that didn't respond to standard drugs. This has not only demonstrated that it can be safely used, it has also provided a great deal of information and helpful tips on the implementation of this diet.

* * * * * * * * *

The idea of metabolic therapies for cancer has been around for many years. The first published account of the effect of dietary manipulation, on the growth of human brain tumors, was published in 1995 by Linda Nebeling, et al.[3, 4] She reported that the use of a ketogenic diet in two children with brain tumors reduced glucose use by the tumor cells. In fact, this pilot study showed the utility of a ketogenic diet in these patients. Since that time there has been one trial for advanced cancer patients,[5] a published case report[6] and numerous anecdotal reports[7] describing the use of alterations in metabolism for the treatment of cancer.

In addition, Dr. Thomas Seyfried, one of the pioneers of metabolic therapy for the treatment of cancer, began to demonstrate the beneficial effects of calorie restriction and a ketogenic diet on tumor growth in a number of mouse models of brain tumors. This work also began to define some of the antitumor effects of altering metabolism by reducing glucose and increasing ketones, mostly through caloric restriction; that is, severely reducing the amount of food provided. For a number of years, the antitumor effects of the ketogenic diet were thought to be primarily due to the reduction in blood glucose.

My laboratory's entry into this field began with an experiment using tumor cells grown in the lab. We added ketones to cells grown under conditions of high glucose, and we found that simply adding ketones slowed the growth of these tumor cells. Furthermore, if we added a chemotherapy agent the effect was even more pronounced.[8]

We then began studying the effects of a ketogenic diet in a mouse model of brain tumors. This work showed that the expression of many different genes, not only those involved in metabolism, was altered in tumor cells from mice given the ketogenic diet. Furthermore, the effects were different in the tumor than they were in the normal brain.[9]

We also tested the effect of a ketogenic diet in combination with radiation therapy in our model.[10] The animals given the two therapies together not only survived longer, the tumor actually disappeared in nine of eleven animals! Again, when we tried ketones and radiation on cells grown in the laboratory we saw a reduction in growth, even in the presence of high levels of glucose.

We have since done a number of studies to identify how the ketogenic diet may be helping to fight the tumor in combination with radiation, or alone. We found that when a ketogenic diet is given, even without restricting the amount that can be eaten (calorie restriction): the tumors have reduced blood vessel formation; there is reduced swelling around the tumor; reduced inflammation (even after radiation treatment); and reduced production of growth factors that typically promote tumor growth.

This work, in addition to the work we have done on cells grown in the laboratory and work done by our colleagues, shows that altering metabolism has many effects on cancer cells. Not only are we slowing their growth by reducing glucose (and thus reducing the energy available to them), we are also altering a variety of processes in these cells. Some of these effects are likely due to ketones alone, some are likely due to the reduction in glucose, and some are likely due to a combination of the two.

The effects of the ketogenic diet are varied, and complementary to the anti-tumor effects of standard therapies such as radiation and chemotherapy. We believe that combining the ketogenic diet with other therapies may be a non-toxic way to enhance the anti-tumor effects of both, thus providing a "one-two punch" to the cancer cells.

* * * * * * * * *

So, with all of this positive data, why has this therapy not been embraced by oncology physicians? There are probably many reasons. Comments we have heard include: "It is too difficult to follow," "It will reduce quality of life," "Patients will lose weight," etc. In fact, these criticisms have some value. The ketogenic diet is not for everyone. It is a challenge to follow and requires that patients and their caregivers change the way they prepare meals. Food is not just nutrition in our society; it is a social event and is typically the center of interactions with friends and families. Thus, changing a cancer patient's diet can impact quality of life in some ways. However, we have also been told that patients like the fact that this is something *they* can do to fight their disease. Most therapies are done *to* them by healthcare professionals. This can lead to a feeling of helplessness for the patient and their loved ones. The ketogenic diet allows them to actively participate in fighting their disease, and monitoring their blood glucose and ketone levels provides them with positive reinforcement.

Weight loss is another common concern among cancer physicians. Although not as common in brain tumor patients, cancer patients can experience weight loss due to cachexia, often in the end stages of their disease. This type of weight loss is a result of muscle atrophy or muscle "wasting" and is not the same as the weight loss that can occur from a ketogenic diet. The ketogenic diet promotes the loss of weight from fat, and weight loss due to the ketogenic diet may in fact help *prevent* cachexia, thus helping to improve overall health.[11]

As more information has become available to the public regarding the anti-cancer utility of the ketogenic diet, and its mechanisms of action, there has been an increase in interest from cancer patients. As patients decide to use the ketogenic diet, they are finding more ways to make it a bit easier, such as working with a chef at a local restaurant so they can go out for a celebratory dinner with their family, finding ways to package meals, and having group cooking days, etc.

Foundations such as the Charlie Foundation and Matthew's Friends have wonderful web sites with recipes and tips to make the diet more user-friendly.

Finally, the success of pioneer patients, such as Mindy Elwell, is showing the medical community there is a place for this type of therapy in the treatment of cancer, particularly brain tumors. We are seeing a slow change in attitude that has led to the recent opening of clinical trials to study the utility of this approach for brain tumors and other cancers.[12] The results of these trials will provide further impetus for the use of metabolic therapies for the treatment of cancer.

Reference List

1. *Warburg O, Wind F, Negelein E. The metabolism of tumors in the body. J Gen Physiol 1927;8:519-30.*

2. *Warburg O. On the origin of cancer cells. Science 1956;123:309-14.*

3. *Nebeling LC, Lerner E. Implementing a ketogenic diet based on medium-chain triglyceride oil in pediatric patients with cancer. J Am Diet Assoc 1995;95:693-7.*

4. *Nebeling LC, Miraldi F, Shurin SB, Lerner E. Effects of a ketogenic diet on tumor metabolism and nutritional status in pediatric oncology patients: two case reports. J Am Coll Nutr 1995;14:202-8.*

5. *Rieger J, Bahr O, Maurer GD, Hattingen E, Franz K, Brucker D, et al. ERGO: a pilot study of ketogenic diet in recurrent glioblastoma. Int J Oncol 2014;44:1843-52.*

6. *Zuccoli G, Marcello N, Pisanello A, Servadei F, Vaccaro S, Mukherjee P, et al. Metabolic management of glioblastoma multiforme using standard therapy together with a restricted ketogenic diet: Case Report. Nutrition and Metabolism 2010;7:33-53.*

7. Seyfried TN, Shelton LM. Cancer as a metabolic disease. Nutr Metab (Lond) 2010;7:7.:7.

8. Scheck AC, Abdelwahab MG, Fenton K, Stafford P. The ketogenic diet for the treatment of glioma: Insights from genetic profiling. Epilepsy Research 2012;100:327-37.

9. Stafford P, Abdelwahab MG, Kim DY, Preul MC, Rho JM, Scheck AC. The ketogenic diet reverses gene expression patterns and reduces reactive oxygen species levels when used as an adjuvant therapy for glioma. Nutr Metab (Lond) 2010;7:74.

10. Abdelwahab MG, Fenton KE, Preul MC, Rho JM, Lynch A, Stafford P, et al. The ketogenic diet is an effective adjuvant to radiation therapy for the treatment of malignant glioma. PLoS ONE 2012;7:e36197.

11. Shukla SK, Gebregiworgis T, Purohit V, Chaika NV, Gunda V, Radhakrishnan P, et al. Metabolic reprogramming induced by ketone bodies diminishes pancreatic cancer cachexia. Cancer Metab 2014;2:18.

12. https://clinicaltrials.gov/ct2/results?term=ketogenic+diet+and+cancer& Search=Search

CHAPTER 3

WHAT IS THE KETOGENIC DIET? A REGISTERED DIETICIAN'S POINT OF VIEW

Leonora Renda, RDN
St. Joseph's Hospital and Medical Center
Phoenix, Arizona

Technically Speaking

The Ketogenic Diet provides a high fat, low carbohydrate diet that alters the body's metabolism by increasing the level of *ketones* in the blood while reducing *glucose* and inducing *ketosis*. The liver uses fatty acids to produce ketone bodies, used as fuel for the body—especially, the brain and the heart.

The ketogenic diet has been used to treat seizure disorders since the 1920s. It has also been used to reduce adult obesity, and treat refractory pediatric epilepsy, and adult epilepsy. This diet is best administered under the care of a neurologist and a registered dietitian. It also requires a pre-laboratory evaluation to establish a baseline of blood levels and to monitor glucose and ketone levels.

The *ketogenic ratio* refers to the ratio of fat grams to the combined grams of protein and carbohydrates. In a 4:1 ratio, 1,000 kcal diet, 8 grams of carbohydrates are allowed; 3:1 ratio diet, 16 grams of carbohydrates are allowed; 2:1 diet, 30 grams of carbohydrates are allowed; and in a 1:1 ratio diet, 40-60 grams of carbohydrates are allowed. To help manage the diet, a specific formula called *KetoCal*, a commercial formula with a 4:1 ratio of fat to carbohydrate and protein can be used for the diet.

The *classic ketogenic diet* is an individualized and structured meal plan based on the needs of the patient. Special meal plans are provided, with all foods weighed and eaten in their entirely for best results. This diet requires supervision from a Registered Dietitian Nutritionist who has expertise in managing a ketogenic regimen.

Nutritional Guidelines

A ketogenic diet emphasizes foods rich in natural fats and adequate in protein while restricting foods high in carbohydrates (sugars and starches). Examples of a typical meal include: a source of natural fats (coconut oil, olive oil, cream, butter); a small amount of protein (eggs, chicken breast, 70% lean beef, fish); and some green, leafy vegetables.

How does a Ketogenic Diet work?

Carbohydrates, when eaten, are broken down into glucose (sugar) in the body. The greater the amount of carbohydrates eaten the higher the level of sugar in the body, resulting in higher blood sugar levels. Less carbohydrates, along with more fats and protein, causes the body to actually use stored fat for fuel, instead of sugar. This use of stored fat produces ketones in the body. As your body uses fat for fuel, the ketone level rises and the sugar level decreases.

Why do we control both carbohydrates and proteins?

The body can make glucose from stored glycogen found in the liver, which comes from carbohydrates. The body stores glucose (sugar) when it is not needed for energy. This stored glucose must be depleted to go into ketosis. Protein can also be converted to glucose if needed, for brain function. Excess protein is stored as glycogen, which can keep the body from reaching ketosis.

Is the diet healthy?

The diet alone does not contain enough vitamins and minerals. A daily multiple vitamin and mineral should be taken. You should also drink adequate water, at least a half-gallon daily.

Will I lose weight on the diet?

The ketogenic diet is calculated based on your specific calorie level, what is necessary to maintain your weight. The dietitian will closely monitor your weight and adjust your diet, as needed.

What happens if I cheat on my diet?

You will need to test your ketones and glucose levels daily. If you are not following the meal plans completely, your ketone levels will decrease and your glucose levels will rise. In order to get back into ketosis you may have to reduce your calorie intake until you are back in ketosis.

Will the diet cause high cholesterol?

Most people do not develop high cholesterol on this diet. If you currently have high cholesterol, your diet will revolve around healthy fats.

Sources:

- The Ketogenic Diet, Academy of Nutrition and Dietetic Pediatric Manual, 2007
- Introducing the diet, The Charlie Foundation, http://www.charliefoundation org/explore-ketogenic-diet/explore-1/introducing-the-diet, Jan 2015.

CHAPTER 4

PLANNING A KETOGENIC REGIMEN

Leonora Renda, RDN
St. Joseph's Hospital and Medical Center
Phoenix, Arizona

Ketogenic Diet Guidelines

These guidelines are intended to optimize nutrition while on the 4:1 ketogenic diet, as discussed in the previous chapter. Therefore, it is extremely important to ensure that the foods and liquids are eaten together at each meal, in their entirety, in order to maintain ketosis. Duration on the diet will be determined by the attending Registered Dietitian, Nutritionist (RDN), usually 8-10 weeks (one week before beginning cancer treatment and 2- 4 weeks post-treatment).

General Ketosis Guidelines

You will need:
- Scale to measure food by the gram
- Spatula
- Urine Ketone strips

Limit/avoid:

All grains and carbohydrates: bread, cereal, grains, rice, pasta, potato, corn, green peas, sugar.

Do include:
- Multivitamin with minerals
- Water to help relieve any constipation
- High fiber vegetables such as lettuce, broccoli, cauliflower
- Foods high in fat such as heavy cream, avocado, butter or margarine, mayo and olive oil
- Eat three meals a day

Pre-operative Ketogenic Nutritional Guidelines
(1 week prior to treatment)

Initial caloric intake will be determined by patient's resting energy expenditure, which will be established by the RDN. The purpose of the diet is to create ketosis in the body. Carbohydrates are limited to 10g/day.

Shopping List:
- Gram scale
- Precision Xtra Glucose Ketone monitor with strips
- Urine ketone strips
- Multivitamin with minerals
- Non-starchy vegetables such as cauliflower, broccoli, and lettuce
- Foods high in fats such as heavy cream (36% - 40% butterfat), avocado, butter/margarine, mayo and olive oil, Ghee, coconut oil
- Proteins high in fat such as eggs, bacon, 70% fat beef, nuts
- Other proteins rich foods such as fish, chicken, turkey
- Free foods such as artificial sweeteners, extracts and flavorings, herbs and spices, lemon

Special instructions:
1. Drink at least ½ gallon of water daily
2. Take a multivitamin daily
3. Eat 100% of meals
4. Test ketosis and glucose levels daily

Ketogenic Diet Nutritional Guidelines
Stage, Timeline, Nutrition Recommendations

1   Pre-procedure
1 week prior
- Pretreatment radiation/chemo therapy guidelines
- KetoCal
- Calories to initiate the diet are reduced to the resting energy expenditure of the patient and carbohydrates are limited to 10g/day
- Drink a minimum of water (½ gallon a day)
- Multi-vitamin with minerals
- The classic ketogenic diet consists of a 4:1 ratio of fats to protein and carbohydrates.
- Patient will have daily contact with RDN to report ketosis and glucose levels and to monitor diet.
- Heavy cream, butter and vegetable oils provide the necessary fat.
- Eliminate all sweets, breads, potatoes, rice cereal and pasta.
- All foods must be measured on a gram scale and carefully prepared.
- For the diet to be most effective, 100% of the meal must be eaten.

2   During radiation/chemo therapy
- Meal plans as directed by Registered Dietitian Nutritionist (RDN).
- Calories are based on the total energy expenditure of the patient and carbohydrates are limited to 10-20g/day
- Drink a minimum of water, half-gallon per day

- Multi-vitamin with minerals
- The classic ketogenic diet consists of a 4:1 ratio of fats to protein and carbohydrate.
- Patient will have daily contact with RDN to report ketosis and glucose levels and to monitor diet.
- Heavy cream, butter and vegetable oils provide the necessary fat.
- Eliminate all sweets, breads, potatoes, rice, cereal, and pasta.
- All foods must be measured on a gram scale and carefully prepared.
- For the diet to be most effective, 100% of the meal must be eaten.
- Meal plans will consist of three meals a day with snacks as needed.
- Over the counter medications might be needed for constipation.

A typical meal is composed of a small amount of fruit and/or vegetables, protein rich food with the majority consisting of a source of fat such as butter, vegetable oil, heavy cream, avocado and mayo.

3 Post-procedure
- Continue with diet for 2- 4 weeks as directed by Physician and Registered Dietitian
- Transition to a Modified Atkins (Keto) diet

Fat Tips
The majority of calories in the ketogenic diet come from fat. The following are some ways to incorporate fat into meals. Use only the amounts of fat calculated for your diet.

Butter, coconut oil* or margarine
- Reheat cooked meat in butter in small pan. The butter will absorb into meat.
- Melt butter, add a pinch of cinnamon and a few drops of liquid saccharine. Serve in a small cup as a drink.

- Melt some butter, pour into ice-cube mold. Weigh out portion size to eat.
- Mix melted butter into applesauce, and then add a pinch of cinnamon and a few drops of liquid saccharine sweetener.
- In a blender, mix melted butter with chopped peaches. Add a few drops of liquid saccharin sweetener and vanilla extract. Freeze the mixture in a small container.
- Mix a pinch of herb into 2-3 tablespoons of softened butter. Refrigerate the mixture for up to 3 days to maximize flavor. Use in meals to enhance the flavor of vegetables or meat.
- Mix butter into peanut butter or softened cream cheese.

Mayonnaise
- Mix mayonnaise with a small amount of cream. Add a pinch of dill weed and salt to make a salad dressing.
- Mix mayonnaise into chopped meats such as chicken, turkey or pork.
- Make egg salad or tuna salad with mayonnaise. Serve with carrot or celery sticks.

Vegetable oils
- Blend oil into mayonnaise. Mix into finely chopped chicken, turkey or tuna.
- Blend some or all of the oil into cream.

*Coconut oil is the natural oil that has been squeezed from the inside of the coconut. It has the highest concentration of medium chain triglycerides (MCTs) of all foods. Medium chain triglycerides are very beneficial for the ketogenic diet since they are easily absorbed into the gut and into the cells. This special fat does not require carnitine like other fats and it also is better in producing ketones than other fats. Coconut oil is prepared in solid form and may be used in the same way that butter is used.

Grade A Heavy Whipping Cream

The butterfat content of the cream should be either 36% or 40%. The label on the carton may not show these percentages. Buy cream that matches the labels shown. Your dietitian will calculate meals with the type of cream that you are able to locate. Check the freshness date on the cream before buying it. Avoid creams containing polysorbate or ingredients ending in "-ose".

For 36% Cream	**For 40% Cream**
Nutrition Facts	Nutrition Facts
Serving size:	Serving size:
½ fluid ounces (15mL)	½ fluid ounces (15mL)
Amount per serving	Amount per serving
Calories: 50	Calories: 60
Calories from fat: 50	Calories from fat: 55
Total fat: 5 grams	Total fat: 6 grams
Total carbohydrate: 0 (or 1g)	Total Carbohydrate: 0 (or 1g)
Protein: 0 grams	Protein: 0 grams

Tips for mixing cream:

Note: Use only the amount allotted. For recipes with whipped cream, weigh the cream after it has been whipped.

- Mix whipped cream and a few drops of pure extract and sweetener. Can be frozen, eaten with a spoon.
- Mix the cream with water to make it taste more like milk.
- Mix the cream with 5 drops of pure vanilla or chocolate extract. Mix with water or diet caffeine-free club soda.

- Make a "cream soda" by mixing the cream with diet, caffeine-free soda such as root beer.
- Mix whipped cream with allotted fruit (chopped). Eat with a spoon.
- Make sherbet by whipping cream into sugar-free Jell-O® (must be calculated) that is just about gelled. Serve frozen.
- Make "hot chocolate" by adding unsweetened baking chocolate (must be calculated) or pure chocolate extract (free food). Heat till warm.
- Add sour cream to whipped cream (from a calculated recipe). Add chopped fruit. Tastes like yogurt.

Free Foods

"Free foods" are foods that have little or no calories or they contain mostly fat calories. These foods are included to make meals more interesting. Some are limited to amounts shown.

Extracts and flavorings: Up to 15 drops can be used in one day. Imitation or pure extracts may be consumed.

Some examples are:
- Bickford™
- Flavorings, McCormick™
- Durkee™
- DaVinci Gourmet Sugar-Free Syrups

Sweeteners: Must be calorie and carbohydrate free
- Liquid Saccharine products: Sweet'N Low®, Sweet 10
- Stevia powders or liquids: Stevita™
- Necta Sweet™ ¼ grain saccharin tablets that can be dissolved in water

Beverages: Give beverages in the amounts recommended by RDN
- Water or ice chips

- Water sweetened with the above sweeteners
- Flavored bottled water beverages that are caffeine, carbohydrate and calorie free

Nonstick cooking sprays: Ingredient list should include a vegetable oil only.

One of the following may be eaten each day. Additional amounts need to be calculated into your meals.
- 25 grams lettuce
- 3 small (ripe) black olives
- 1 black walnut
- 1 macadamia nut
- 1 pecan
- 3 hazelnuts (filberts)

Herbs and spices: Use just a pinch for flavor. Salt may be used as desired for seasoning.
- Pepper, basil, oregano, dill or other pure herbs
- Cinnamon, nutmeg or other pure spices

Prepared by The Charlie Foundation
Fruit and Vegetable List for the Ketogenic Diet

Fruit or juice: fresh, frozen or canned without sugar. Do not use dried fruit.

10%
(Use amount prescribed)

Applesauce *(unsweetened)*	Apricot	Blackberries
Cantaloupe	Grapefruit	Guava
Honeydew Melon	Kiwi	Mango
Nectarine	Orange	Papaya
Peaches	Pineapple	Raspberries
Strawberries	Tangerine	Watermelon

15%
(Use 2/3 amount prescribed)

Apple *(with skin)*	Blueberries	Cherries *(sweet/sour)*
Grapes	Pears	Plums

Vegetables: Fresh, canned or frozen. Measure raw (R) or cooked (C) as specified.

Group A
(Use twice amount specified)

Asparagus/C	Beet greens/C	Cabbage/C
Celery/R or C	Chicory/C	Cucumbers/C
Eggplant/C	Endive/R	Green pepper/R or C
Poke/C	Radish/R	Rhubarb/R
Sauerkraut/C	Summer Squash/C	Swiss Chard/C
Tomato/R	Tomato juice	Turnips/C
Turnip greens/C	Watercress/R	

Group B
(Use amount specified)

Beets/C	Broccoli/C	Brussels sprouts/C
Cabbage/R	Carrots/R or C	Cauliflower/C
Collard greens/C	Dandelion greens/C	Green beans/C
Kale/C	Kohirabi/C	Mushroom/R
Mustard greens/C	Okra/C	Onion/R or C
Rutabaga/C	Spinach/C	Tomato/C
Winter squash/C		

Prepared by The Charlie Foundation
Meal Plans for 2000 calorie diet examples

Cream/Fruit
21 grams	10% Fruit
24 grams	Cream, 50 calories fat
Mix together	

Bacon/Fruit
56 grams	Cream, 36% fat
13 grams	10% Fruit
36 grams	Bacon, cooked crisp – Oscar Mayer
32 grams	Oil, Canola
Mix oil into cream	

Egg/Vegetable
55 grams	Cream, 36% fat
24 grams	Group B Vegetable
94 grams	Egg (raw, mixed well)
47 grams	Butter

Instructions: 1. Melt butter in pan, add vegetables to butter

2. Sautee till vegetables are soft, add eggs

3. Continue cooking till done

Eggs Benedict

55 grams	Cream, 36% fat
48 grams	Butter
14 grams	Bacon, Canadian – Oscar Mayer
60 grams	Egg (raw, mixed well)
5 grams	Cheese, Kraft Deli Deluxe Amer (Pro 4, Fat 7 Carb 0)
15 grams	10% Fruit

Instructions: 1. Mix the cream into mixed egg

2. Mix in melted butter

3. Pour into small fry pan

4. Scramble eggs

5. Serve eggs on Canadian bacon

6. Top with shredded cheese

7. Serve with fruit

Beef Pattie/fruit/Jell-0®

90 grams	Cream, 50 calories fat
17 grams	10% fruit
30 grams	Gelatin, Jell-O® sugar free, prepared
52 grams	Beef, ground 70% lean - cooked
15 grams	Oil, Canola
22 grams	Cream cheese, Organic Valley

Instructions: Pan fry in oil spray or grill ground beef patty

Weigh after cooking

Egg Salad/Vegetable

46 grams	Cream, 50 calories fat
24 grams	Group B Vegetables
10 grams	Egg Yolk – cooked
110 grams	Egg White – cooked
50 grams	Mayonnaise/Hellman's Best Foods
5 grams	Oil, Canola

Instructions:
1. Separate egg white from yolk and chop into fine pieces
2. Weigh cooked egg white and egg yolk separately
3. Mix mayonnaise, egg white and egg yolk together
4. Add a pinch of salt
5. Refrigerate to allow fat to absorb into eggs
6. Mix oil into cream

Chicken Breast/Fruit/Mayo

55 grams	Cream, 36% fat
17 grams	10% Fruit
39 grams	Chicken breast, no skin – cooked
5 grams	Oil, Canola
51 grams	Mayonnaise, Hellmann's Best Foods

Mix cream and fruit together

Avocado snack

65 grams	Avocado

Sample Patient Menu

Breakfast
Choice of 1
2 scrambled eggs with 3 strips of bacon
2 hardboiled eggs with 3 strips of bacon

Lunch - Choice of 1

Chicken and Vegetable #26
1 serving broccoli
1 lemon cut into wedges
3 strips bacon
2 packs mayo, Heinz®
40 gm ghee

Chicken with Lettuce #32
2 servings chicken
100 g romaine lettuce
1 lemon cut into wedges
150 heavy cream, whipped
40 gm ghee

Salad Chop Style #36
120 gm heavy cream whipped
1 lemon, cut into wedges
3 strips soft bacon
2 serving chicken breast
20 gm olives, black
40 gm ghee

Turkey and Vegetable #33
2 serving turkey breast
1 lemon, wedged
1 lemon, wedged
100 gm romaine lettuce
40 gm ghee

Turkey and Vegetable #27
180 gm heavy cream whipped
1 serving steamed broccoli
1 lemon, wedged
2 servings turkey breast
40 gm ghee

Cod with Vegetable no cream #15
90 gm lettuce, romaine
1 lemon, wedged
2 servings baked cod
2 packs mayo
40 gm ghee

Basa with Salad and Cream #22
2 servings Basa (fish)
150 gm heavy cream whipped
90 gm lettuce, romaine
1 lemon, wedged
4 packets mayo

Egg Salad with Salad and Cream #38
4 hard-boiled eggs
150 gm heavy cream whipped
90 gm lettuce, romaine
1 lemon, wedged

Tuna Salad with Salad and Cream #39
4 oz tuna, drained water packed
150 gm heavy cream whipped
90 gm lettuce, romaine
1 lemon, wedged
4 packets mayo

Dinner - Choice of 1

Chicken and Vegetable #26
1 serving broccoli
1 lemon cut into wedges
3 strips bacon
2 packs mayo, Heinz®
40 gm ghee

Turkey and Vegetable #33
2 serving turkey breast
1 lemon, wedged
1 lemon, wedged
100 gm romaine lettuce
40 gm ghee

Chicken with Lettuce #32
2 servings chicken
100 g romaine lettuce
1 lemon cut into wedges
150 heavy cream, whipped
40 gm ghee

Turkey and Vegetable #27
180 gm heavy cream whipped
1 serving steamed broccoli
1 lemon, wedged
2 servings turkey breast
40 gm ghee

Salad Chop Style #36
120 gm heavy cream whipped
1 lemon, cut into wedges
3 strips soft bacon
2 serving chicken breast
20 gm olives, black
40 gm ghee

Basa with Salad and Cream #22
2 servings Basa
150 gm heavy cream whipped
90 gm lettuce, romaine
1 lemon, wedged
40 gm ghee
40 gm ghee

Tuna Salad with Salad and Cream #39
4 oz tuna, drained water packed
150 gm heavy cream whipped
90 gm lettuce, romaine
1 lemon, wedged
4 packets mayo
40 gm ghee

Cod with Vegetable no cream #15
90 gm lettuce, romaine
1 lemon, wedged
2 servings baked cod
2 packs mayo
40 gm ghee

Egg Salad with Salad and Cream #38
4 hard-boiled eggs
150 gm heavy cream whipped
90 gm lettuce, romaine
1 lemon, wedged
4 packets mayo

CHAPTER 5

MY RESPONSE TO CANCER: STARVE!

The type of tumor I have is very aggressive. There are no treatments, surgeries or diets that can guarantee survival or reverse the effects of anaplastic astrocytoma. It is a beast. After my craniotomy in March 2014, the doctors warned us that there could be some rogue cancer cells hanging around, necessitating more radiation and chemotherapy. I agreed to do what they recommended and also dove right back into the KD after I recovered from the surgery. At this point, the KD was the only tool in my belt. If something else comes along in the way of a gentle medication I will consider it. But I will not do another round of radiation. I believe I lost too much of my brain function.

So, at this stage, I choose to starve any remaining cancer cells in my body. Let them suffer. I'm doing fine, considering. I continue to enjoy eating the KD way. It feels clean and simple. We use basic ingredients, no tricks, nothing artificial and—best of all—nothing complicated. After eating my meals, I'm full and satisfied. There's variety and flavor in what I eat. Eating is supposed to be pleasurable, and the KD meals are delicious and satisfying; thus, keeping me feeling positive about the way we are pushing this thing down.

During the initial stages of embracing the KD, I was very excited and positive because I had so much support; I just knew I would make a go of it. I didn't have any physical feelings of withdrawal from sugar or carbs. I just kept filling my body with healthy stuff and lots of water and sunlight. I surrounded myself with positive people and positive activities. Physically, I was feeling fine, with no headaches or other symptoms. I was exercising and carrying on my normal stay-at-home mom routine. Another way of knowing I was succeeding with the KD was testing my blood and urine. It was like getting a good report card.

I did fall off the KD wagon, though. It was on my birthday in 2013, when somebody insisted I have a piece of cake. I had a slice, and the next thing I knew, I had a piece of Halloween candy, and then pumpkin pie at Thanksgiving, and cheesecake at Christmas, and so on—it's that easy to fall out of the KD routine. Sugars are like an addictive drug! Also, I became over-confident. I was doing well and thought I was over the hump. During those months, I noticed my left side was getting weaker, especially my leg. Rich noticed that when I smiled, my smile was crooked, and I detected some speech anomalies. I wasn't very excited for my next scan. I had a strong suspicion there would be some growth, some areas of concern. And there were. From that point, my response to cancer became one word: STARVE!

* * * * * * * * *

When looking at the cause and effect regarding the elimination of sugar and processed foods, it became clear to me there's a direct connection between skin condition and nutrition. One great example of "you are what you eat," is seeing the effects of a clean KD on my skin. I've struggled with acne since I was thirteen years old. I tried various means of resolving that embarrassing problem, from creams to masks to antibiotics. Nothing worked. The school of thought I grew up with was, there's no correlation between food and acne. This unfortunate belief let me off the hook, "Eat what you want, it doesn't matter." After being on the KD for about two months, I realized it did matter. My face cleared up within weeks of changing my nutrition. At the same time, I noticed my fingernails were no longer cracking, peeling, and breaking. Throughout my cancer journey, I've been told that my skin looks healthy and my eyes are bright and glowing. I believe that the elimination of processed foods, sugar and low carbohydrates contributed to this. You truly are what you eat.

Aside from looking and feeling good, you will appreciate having little or no cravings for processed foods, sugar and carbs. It will probably take a week or two for you to get over the pull toward the foods you're accustomed to. Once they're out of your system, avoiding taboo foods will be much easier. You may have headaches in the first couple of days; stay well hydrated, get adequate sleep, exercise and sunshine. Enlist the help and support of your family and friends. Ask that they respectfully keep an eye on you and that they refrain from offering foods that are off limits. Of course, you need to police yourself and be responsible for your actions and choices. But it doesn't hurt to have consistent, sincere and loving support from family and friends.

As far as seeing immediate results, don't be discouraged if you don't get into ketosis immediately; it takes between two and seven days depending on your level of activity, what you're eating and your body type. The state of ketosis can be achieved more quickly if you fast for a day or two and drink lots of water or plain tea with a squeeze of lemon. The best way to do the KD is under the guidance of a registered dietician, especially if you're undergoing cancer therapy.

Tip: By plain tea, I mean unflavored and not decaf. There are carbs in flavored teas, such as vanilla or raspberry, for example.

Eating healthy foods will also keep you feeling fuller longer. I found that when I was full, I didn't care so much about tempting snacks. I could be around all sorts of snacks and treats and be just fine. It's the same principle as not going food shopping on an empty stomach. Ending my addiction to sugar and carbs led me to feel proud and capable. Do I still get cravings? Close friends and family know how much I enjoy desserts and sweets. In the early days of my KD learning curve, I turned to sugar-free Jell-O® to get me through. While I wasn't comfortable consuming artificial colors and other unknown ingredients, that stuff truly saved me during many evenings when I was feeling deprived and restless—and when the kids were having ice cream. The sugar-free Jell-O® helped me over the craving hump. It's not filling, but it *is* sweet, and that's what I was craving—sweet.

* * * * * * * * *

While getting your body *into* ketosis might take a week or two, it sure doesn't take much to fall *out* of ketosis. One night Rich made his famous Brussels sprouts with coconut milk and pineapple. I didn't realize how much pineapple was mixed in until I checked my glucose the next day and it was 139. Yikes!

When eating meals prepared by others, don't hesitate to ask about ingredients. Common sense will be your guide once you get the hang of it. When eating out at a chain restaurant, install a carb content app on your phone before ordering. Our kids checked for carb content of the onion ring stack at Red Robin and we were shocked at what we learned. Some foods have different carb counts when eaten cooked versus raw. Two examples are mushrooms and tomatoes, both of which have lower carbs when eaten raw versus cooked. On the KD, every carb counts.

When reading labels, don't get tripped up by the terms "fat free" and "low fat." These products are usually high in carbs. Your vitamins and supplements may also have carbs that count toward your daily carb max. Your dietitian will work with you to determine what that number is. You'll also need to know the maximum number of daily calories allowed. During the first few weeks, that might be 10-15 grams of carbs per day. This calorie allotment is determined by height and weight. As you move forward and your body starts to consistently produce ketones, your daily carb count may be increased.

Do *not* make this determination on your own. I remember being so excited when I could eat between 30 and 50 grams of carbs per day but still, I kept my carbs as low as possible, figuring, if I'm full, I don't need to worry about it. Your dietitian will work closely with you to determine when your carbs can be increased and this will feel like a reward. Although you still need to eat the right foods, one day you could choose to have a piece of whole wheat toast with butter or natural peanut butter, for instance, as a treat. Just be careful to count the carbs of your "treat," and don't get too comfortable. As I said earlier, you can fall off the wagon very easily. The occasional piece of bread should only be enjoyed once you're fully into ketosis. This small act can preserve your sanity, and you can plan out something to look forward to.

There might be occasions when well-meaning friends and relatives will push foods on you, insisting that you *must* have "just one bite." There will be people who will try to discourage you, and make fun of your diet. Try to explain it to them so they can be on board with you. Absolutely *do not* let this get to you. But be prepared. Think about some snappy comebacks and effective responses. Try them out and make a mental note of which ones worked to put an end to the commentary. Avoid the Debbie Downers in your circles whenever possible.

* * * * * * * * *

The biggest obstacle I faced was staying on track while traveling, even on short day trips. I decided to keep a small, soft cooler packed with some of my essentials in spice containers: coconut oil; chia seeds (ground fine in a coffee bean grinder); and high-quality cinnamon (for flavoring meals and drinks). These items only make sense to bring along if you will be able to have a hand in preparing your own meals, such as at a friend's house, but it's good to get into the habit of bringing your own "customization" ingredients, just in case. Once you get to your destination, have access to a fridge and, hopefully, a kitchen, you can pick up heavy cream, eggs, butter, avocados and other items that will help keep your fat levels up. My sister-in-law often picks up coconut oil, flax seed oil and apple cider vinegar before we arrive for visits. It's a kind and convenient gesture.

Once I got into a familiar routine with the proper foods and such, traveling and going out to dinner became more comfortable. It's really not that hard to abide by the diet once you learn about your options. For example, it's not difficult to keep a stash of nuts on hand while traveling; they keep for a long time, are satisfying and filling. Macadamia nuts are among my favorites and their high fat content fits the KD bill quite well. I have a whole list of food choices, and even personal recipes, in the next chapter.

Going out to dinner was a big challenge and a bit uncomfortable, at first. The delectable dishes at most restaurants are rich in carbs and sugars. Again, it's not impossible to learn how to maneuver through a dinner out, once you get used to customizing your options, something most restaurants will accommodate, as far as substitutions anyway, such as replacing starches with veggies or salad.

There's a whole list of recommended food choices, as well as those to avoid in the next chapter, but with regard to dinner out, I mostly gravitated toward salads, always a good option, but avoided raisins and croutons. Once you learn more about hidden sugars in most foods, you'll realize the devil is in the details, such as salad dressings (most of the commercial brands you buy at the store are loaded with sugar). I stick to balsamic vinegar or fresh lemon juice, even in restaurants, and steer clear of the salad buffet (lots of temptation there, as well as sugar-loaded salad dressings).

On occasion, when preparing for a meal out, I would actually eat my ketogenic dinner before hand. Our dinner companions would understand that I was full (which was true) and that I might pick at some veggies or a salad. After a while, people around you will begin to respect your KD choice, knowing it might be saving your life or, at the least, improving your condition.

Some tips I discovered from my professional team, and information you should seek if and when you decide to adopt the KD:

- Learn about how the KD works in conjunction with chemotherapy meds
- Learn about how the KD can bring down glucose levels
- Ask about how, when taken concurrently, the KD can help Temodar be more effective
- We were told the most effective time to do the KD is while undergoing radiation. Ask your professionals about that.
- Vigorous exercise can raise blood sugar levels and you should consider walking versus running. Strenuous muscle activity releases lactic acid into the blood, which can be converted into glucose by the liver and released back into the bloodstream.
- Some people may need to begin this diet in a hospital setting for proper monitoring.
- Patients taking steroids need to know that some medications raise blood sugar, and it also may not work if a patient is receiving intravenous medicines that contain glucose. These meds will interfere with carb count and prevent, or throw you out of, ketosis.

CHAPTER 6

MY PERSONAL KETOGENIC TIPS AND FOOD CHOICES

After reading the previous chapters, you get the idea about how the KD works. But I'll give it one more overview, just to put it in my own language, as I understand it. For the layperson, this may be easier to understand. At the very least, it may underscore what you already read.

The KD requires a stringent, but not impossible, adherence to certain foods and a restriction of others: a very low intake of sugars and carbs (~3%); lowered levels of proteins (~7%); and high fat levels (~90%). There's a scientific reason behind these percentages, as Dr. Scheck and Leonora Renda (my RDN advisor) mentioned earlier.

Measuring the amounts of food and the types of food according to the above breakdown, forces the body into starvation mode. We don't actually starve though. The body goes through ketosis, meaning it makes its own energy from what's already in our bodies—fat. Without a decent level of glucose from all the carbs and sugars that were eliminated with the KD, the body begins to make ketones from fat breakdown to replace the glucose it's no longer getting.

This differs from the popular low-carb diets (such as the Atkin's Diet) because protein levels are almost as low as the carbs themselves.

A high protein diet won't allow the body to achieve a real shift in metabolism on a cellular level; one that shifts away from glucose to ketones. The reason for this is because most of the protein (meats) that accompany a low-carb diet tend to have amino acids that can make that protein convert into glucose—sugar. To eliminate as much glucose as possible and really starve those cancer cells, we need to limit our protein intake, as well.

As Dr. Scheck outlined in Chapter 2, our bodies can make ketones out of fat. Almost all the cells in our body can utilize either these ketones *or* glucose for energy. For a cancer cell, however, glucose is the *only* energy it can metabolize. That's because a defect in cancer cells prevents them from being able to absorb ketones. Now you see why it makes sense for cancer patients to minimize sugars. If you can feed all the good cells in your body with ketones but starve the cancer cells by depriving them of glucose—their only source of energy—why wouldn't you try it?

If you're considering the KD to fight your cancer, first talk to your doctor and then meet with the dietitian at your treatment center. Ask him or her for info on KetoCalculator (www.ketocalculator.com), a web site that can help you track your meals. You'll need a special number to become a member. The hospital dietitian can help you develop a menu that's just right for your height and weight and, to some degree, your activity level.

Each time I was about to prepare a meal, I would go on the website and gather the ingredients for the recipe I chose and weigh everything to the gram. My hospital provided me with a product called KetoCal, available in powder or liquid form. It was very helpful for me to have on hand because it's nutritionally balanced with the correct ratio needed for the ketogenic diet. KetoCal is made by a company called Nutricia North America. If you're having trouble-obtaining KetoCal, ask the dietitian or your doctor for a prescription.

One site I found particularly helpful was www. charliefoundation.org It was formed in honor of a boy named Charlie

Abrahams whose parents implemented the KD to successfully control his epileptic seizures. The website has everything you'll need to know in order to get started. You'll also learn how to receive support to implement the diet successfully. Recipes and videos will show you how to prepare the food properly.

Over the past two-plus years that I've been on the KD, I've developed my own basket of goodies. In some recipes, this involves counting out exactly eight blueberries. No kidding. To eliminate any guessing, you can go to a website to find ingredient lists and directions, or ask the dietician for a paper copy of food lists and recipes. On many occasions, these made it much easier for us to consult while shopping at the grocery store.

On a typical day, here's a breakdown of the meals I would eat:

Breakfast
Egg, Vegetables, Cheese, Hot Sauce. Optional: Sour Cream and Bacon.

One egg, prepared in any style you like, topped with sautéed vegetables, cheese, and hot sauce or cayenne pepper. Feel free to add a glob of sour cream and a piece of bacon. It might not sound like this would be enough to fill you up, but it will because of the fat and protein content.

We always keep plenty of eggs on hand. With a flat 1 gram of carbs per egg, it's easy to stay within the right carb count at breakfast time. Be sure to calculate the carb count of any toppings or vegetables you might be having at breakfast time.

Morning Snack
Check the low-carb snack list on the following pages. It's okay to have a snack between breakfast and lunch.

TIP: For an on-the-go lunch or snack, Mix up a KetoCal shake with a quarter-cup berries and coconut oil in the blender. Stock your freezer with frozen berries, just in case your fresh ones spoil.

Lunch

Salad, Lettuce Wrap, or a Shake.

We keep lean turkey and provolone cheese on hand for rolling up in a romaine leaf with mayo for a quick and easy lunch.

Egg salad is also tasty and satisfying. We enjoy it with coarse black pepper, sea salt and chopped romaine. Hard-boiled eggs are a handy low carb snack to keep around. Our kids love them too.

Avocado slices topped with diced tomato or salsa (or any hot sauce), salt, pepper and squeeze of lime. Delicious and filling.

TIP: Mayo gets a bad rap but it's actually a KD staple for us. Steer clear of spreads (Miracle Whip, for example) and any with more than a few ingredients.

Dinner

Fish, pork, chicken or red meat.

Low carb vegetables and a salad, depending on the day's carb and calorie count thus far.

TIP: Always have salad ingredients on hand. Incorporate greens, but be mindful of carb levels. When trying to get into ketosis, every little carb counts.

Keeping my calorie count low and my fat high kept me in steady ketosis. Knowing what to eat and how much to eat sounds like it would be simple but it's risky to simply guess. Start by weighing your foods and, soon, you'll know the basic amounts for each portion. It's a new routine that you'll get accustomed to with a little bit of practice.

TIP: While you're a newbie, it's best to check carb count and keep a record of your meals, at least while you're getting acclimated to your new lifestyle. Consider an app for your phone to help monitor calorie intake and record your levels.

Ketogenic Snacks:

Nuts: Almonds, Brazil Nuts, Macadamia (other nuts are fine too but refer to the Tips below about the other varieties and portion amounts).

Avocado with a squeeze of lime, sea salt and hot sauce.

Veggie burgers with optional toppings: diced tomato, hot sauce, salt, pepper, lime, ricotta cheese.

Olives

Low-Carb Cheeses: Brie, bleu, Parmesan, feta, cheddar, cream cheese.

Kale leaves, drizzled with olive oil, baked on a tray till crisp, top with salt and pepper after cooking.

High-quality, low-carb Chocolate: The following are some brands you can try guilt-free: Ross Chocolates, Russell Stover Chocolates, Atkins Chocolates, Torta Fina Chocolates, Hershey's®, Asher's® Chocolates.

You can satisfy your sweet tooth and not compromise ketosis.

Tuna or Chicken Salad (great for lunch or dinner as well).

Bell Pepper Strips (dip in hummus or bleu cheese dressing, or just plain).

Green tea with Lemon (hot tea in a bag, not the cold soft-drink type).

Romaine Roll-Ups: lean turkey with cheese and mustard or mayonnaise inside a large lettuce leaf; romaine lettuce is highly-nutritious and sturdy.

Cucumber Slices

Celery Sticks with Peanut Butter: check the label on the peanut butter; many popular brands have sugar in them.

* * * * * * * * *

More About Nuts:

The better nuts are *almonds*. A low-carb serving is twelve almonds. They're also great to have chopped so you can sprinkle them over salads and stir-fried vegetables.

Brazil nuts and *macadamia nuts* are also beneficial because they're high in fat content yet low enough in carb content. You can enjoy a quarter-cup. I love their rich, buttery flavor.

Regular peanuts are inferior in nutritional content and they're higher in carbs. I recommend choosing something else when possible.

Cashews are high in carbs but they sure hit the spot. Adherence to the KD is hugely dependent upon staying full and feeling satisfied. Cashews can be a major craving-crusher (salty and satisfying), but watch your intake! We know that one serving is seventeen nuts. We also know they're addictive, so I recommend you do what I do and count them out, put the container out of reach and away from view, and enjoy your seventeen cashews. It's so easy to go overboard.

TIP: Nuts are a great source of protein and fat. But there's a difference among the wide varieties available. They're best in bulk (not pre-packaged), raw and unsalted.

If you must buy canned, read the labels and steer clear of the various hydrogenated oils and sugars.

Cancer-Fighting Food Pairings

While discovering my new and healthy nutrition regimen, I learned about food synergy: food combinations that really optimize health when they're paired up. Here's a list of my favorites:

Tomatoes and Broccoli:

Tomatoes contain lycopene and vitamins C and A. Broccoli contains the cancer fighting photochemicals beta-carotene, isothiocyanates, and indoles.

It's better to eat tomatoes than to take a lycopene supplement. Cooked tomatoes may be better than raw. Chopping and heating make the cancer-fighting constituents of tomatoes and broccoli more active and more easily absorbed.

Tea and Lemon:

Tea is high in antioxidant polyphenols, including catechins (potent cancer fighters) and flavonoids. When lemon is added to green tea, it results in 80% of the catechins to remain after digestion versus only 20% when ingested separately.

I buy Matcha green tea at Costco. It's a great deal with individually wrapped tea bags in quantity. I use a stainless steel Breville kettle to boil water quickly and I'm sure to drink three cups a day. I've found I don't actually enjoy the tea unless I squeeze some lemon into it. It's a great habit.

Kale and Lemon:

Combining the vitamin C from citrus fruits with iron-rich, leafy greens makes the plant-based iron easier to absorb.

Turmeric and black pepper:
Studies show that Turmeric has anti-cancer and anti-inflammatory properties due to its active ingredient Curcumin.

TIP: I keep a glass spice jar filled with a combination of coarse black pepper and Turmeric. I shake it onto eggs, vegetables or soups.

My Pantry Essentials
As I got accustomed to the KD, I started stocking my kitchen with essential items. These are some pantry staples that are great to keep on hand so you can get creative.

Heavy Cream
It's great for keeping up the fat levels; very rich and makes you feel satisfyingly full. I use it in coffee and with eggs. I also add some into the blender when I make smoothies. Another great use is to add some to chicken dishes and mix it with butter and cheese to make sauces. You can even use a little in your vegetable stir fry.

Lemons and Limes
A squeeze of Vitamin C for squeezing into water and tea. Also great for a flavor enhancer to all sorts of meals.

Coconut Oil
Very high in Omega 3's and it really boosts fat content while also adding great flavor. I've found multiple uses.

Almond Milk

For those doing the KD without dairy products, almond milk is a versatile ingredient to keep handy. Mix it in with protein shakes and use it as a substitute for regular milk.

When I first began shopping for what I would need in order to do the KD correctly, I looked into boxed versions of almond and rice milk. But when I read the labels, I realized the list of ingredients included a variety of additives and artificial ingredients. This was disappointing. So I started making my own in a Blendtec blender. See my recipe tip below.

TIP: Make Your Own Almond Milk. It's easy! I use the Blendtec to make all natural almond milk using just two ingredients: Almonds and Water.

Homemade Almond Milk

Ingredients:
4 1/2 cups filtered water
1 cup raw, unsalted almonds, soaked overnight and rinsed

Optional: a few drops of pure, organic vanilla or agave nectar

Measure out one cup almonds, put in blender, cover with filtered water and refrigerate overnight.

Blend until pulverized

If desired, strain the milk through a cheesecloth to remove skins. (I don't mind the skins and I like to keep things simple.). You can spice it up a bit with some drops of vanilla or agave nectar, but plain tastes great too.

TIP: Keep almond milk handy for use in smoothies, soups, in coffee, and as a substitute for regular milk.

Frozen Items To Keep On Hand
Berries
Spinach
Broccoli
Kale (organic if possible)

Herbs
It's easy and inexpensive to grow fresh herbs. If this isn't up your alley, dried herbs are fine. I love the enticing aroma of fresh basil and mint, just to name a couple of stand-outs, that add great flavor to so many dishes.

Buy fresh ginger root at most grocery stores and Asian markets. I store them in the freezer so they keep longer. I've also found they're easier to grate when frozen. This also works well with turmeric root.

Depending on what vegetables you like, here's a listing of low-carb and high-carb vegetables. It's always a good idea to keep some fresh vegetables on hand, for a quick stir fry, raw with a dip, to throw into the blender for a shake, or to roast in the oven, drizzled with oil, lemon, salt and pepper.

Low-Carb Vegetables

Artichokes
Asparagus
Avocado
Bell Peppers
Bok Choy
Broccoli
Brussels Sprouts
Cabbage
Cauliflower
Celery
Chard
Collard Greens
Cucumbers
Eggplant
Fennel
Garlic
Green Beans
Jalapeño Peppers

Kale
Leeks
Lettuce
Mushrooms
Mustard Greens
Okra
Onions
Pumpkin
Radish
Scallions
Snap Peas
Spaghetti Squash
Spinach
Summer Squash
Tomatillos
Tomatoes
Turnips
Zucchini

High-Carb vegetables (starchy):

Beets
Carrots
Corn

Peas
Potatoes
Sweet Potatoes/Yams

Additional Notes

Acquire An Excellent Blender
Having a really good blender makes life so much easier. You'll find it enjoyable tossing ingredients together for effortless smoothies, shakes and green drinks.

Purchase the best blender you can afford. We have the Blendtec. The only downside I've discovered is that the canister isn't recommended for the dishwasher, except on occasion.

I use coconut oil almost daily and I find it hard to remove the film when hand-washing. To preserve the life of your blender, it's best to stay loyal to its warranty and it's instructions. I recommend you rinse immediately after use and fill it with soapy water. Leave it to soak, and that usually makes cleaning effortless.

The competitor of the Blendtec is the Vitamix, comparable in power and price, although the Blendtec is a bit cheaper, and comes with an excellent recipe and suggestion book.

Eat Garlic
Purchase whole heads of garlic, roast with olive oil and pop them in your mouth for a tasty and healthy snack. There are no vampires at our house.

Use Apple Cider Vinegar
Bragg's Organic Apple Cider Vinegar, to be precise. Add a tablespoon or two, to taste, to water or to green drinks daily. It will assist your immune system.

Buy Ketone Test Strips

To determine when you're in ketosis, you'll be able to use either urine test strips or blood ketone test strips. I like the Precision Xtra Meter, but I also use the urine strips occasionally. Both blood and urine test strips are a bit expensive. For example, a box of fifty glucose test strips for the Nova Max® Blood Glucose Monitor will run you about twenty dollars.

If you think you'll have a hard time poking yourself in the finger, you may prefer the urine strips. This may sound silly, but I look forward to the testing because it encourages me, and it's like a pay-off. Also, I admit it's rather cool to see the magenta color creep across the little square on the test urine strips. It means I'm doing it right; it's empowering and rewarding, like acing a test.

Shop around for the meter and the strips to find the best price; they vary according to the retailer. I've found amazon.com to be affordable and convenient.

TIP: A handy feature of using a meter is it maintains a history of your readings so you don't need to write them down. Believe me, you'll appreciate that.

In the beginning, I kept a journal to log everything I ate and to record my sugar/glucose readings, weight and blood pressure. Sometimes I joked that my full-time job was to stay alive; it becomes such a constant and focused mindset. After getting into a routine, however, I no longer need to write everything down. The use of Ketostix (urine test strips), a glucose monitor and my weight will let me know if I'm on or off track.

CHAPTER 7

VITAMINS, SUPPLEMENTS AND HERBS

Supplementation

Each doctor that I spoke to throughout the past couple of years about anything natural for healing responded like this: "There's not enough research on that and the FDA has not approved it."

So it's important to note that I can only describe and explain my own program, what I took and why, with no recommendation for anyone else's specific needs. As a result of an individual's consistency, commitment and faith in its power, supplements can be a major factor in healing. They can also be viewed as an encouraging, proactive process, an important part of your treatment plan.

During the dive into my first round of cancer and nutrition books, I started becoming familiar with various herbs and foods that were referred to as "power foods" and "anti-cancer." One link would lead to another, and the urge for information and knowledge set in. I found reputable sources for ordering what I needed and I learned what to look for as far as seals of approval. My opinion changed regarding stores like Vitamin World and Hi-Health. Before this intense education, it had never occurred to me to investigate the "other" ingredients in Centrum® daily vitamins, which were casually recommended by my neuro-oncologist. "Just go to

Walgreens or CVS and get a store brand Centrum®-type multivitamin," he said. After a little digging into that topic, though, I decided it was an inferior product. I wound up choosing Shaklee-brand vitamins, based on recommendations from a friend, a Shaklee customer for fifteen-plus years and also a believer in supplementation.

Once I had the basics of supplementation down, the more advanced learning progressed. Ideally, I would obtain vitamins through food, but I considered taking other nutrients like turmeric and broccoli sprouts in capsule form, for convenience and for ensuring consistency.

Tip: Take your supplements and vitamins with plenty of water. If possible, have someone with you when you're taking your meds and supplements in case you choke.

Additional Tips

You can purchase a supplement tray at any drugstore, Walmart or amazon.com. I like the one that allows you to take out the container for one day at a time and stick it in your purse, lunchbox or cooler. Choose a day that works for you to fill your pill/supplement tray. I preferred this ritual take place on the weekend, while having coffee or watching the news. I would be thinking about my belief in what the extra nutrients could do. After investing money and time in them, I was sure to take along the day's meds (prescriptions too), so there would be no missing or forgetting doses. The pill tray that we have has each day in a separate, removable section for morning, noon, dinner, and bedtime doses.

These are the supplements that were recommended for me and their recognized benefits. I'm not specifying any dosage because everyone's needs are different.

Hoxsey Formula: Herbal treatment consisting of zinc, bloodroot, licorice, red clover, burdock root and other roots and barks. Check out www.topdocumentaryfilms.com/hoxsey:how healing becomes a crime.

Astralagus Root: Helps stimulate white blood cells and protects against invading organisms. It also enhances production of the important natural compound interferon to fight against viruses.

Broccoli Sprouts: Cancer fighters; contains phytonutrients and antioxidants.

Power Shrooms: Supports immune function.

Vitamin D: Plays a key role in immune function and helps reduce inflammation. I take it daily but it just so happens that living in sunny Arizona contributes naturally to my intake as well.

Green Powder: Add to blender when making smoothies and juices. Contains alfalfa leaf, wheat grass, oat grass, barley grass, parsley, spinach, kale, cilantro, broccoli, and dandelion.

Zinc: Necessary for white blood cell function. It helps wounds heal and helps the immune system fight off bacteria and viruses, as a catalyst in the immune system's killer response to foreign bodies.

Green Tea: Stimulates production of white blood cells. Green tea is most effective when combined with lemon.

Selenium: Vital to the development and movement of white blood cells. Try Brazil nuts, which are high in selenium.

Chia Seeds: The Mayan word for strength. Many benefits: helps with constipation, low calorie, filling, loaded with fiber, protein, Omega

3 fatty acids, and various micronutrients and antioxidants. I like a brand called Mila, but it's out of my budget to afford on a regular basis. Mostly I buy it in the bulk section at our Sprouts store (similar to Whole Foods).

There's an endless list of herbs and supplements you can spend money on without ever truly knowing their effectiveness. If you are serious about supplementation and don't want to waste your money, plan on doing some research and crosschecking.

Tip: Ask around in your health-nut circles for a recommendation to an herbalist. Check credentials. I arranged to have a phone consult with a clinic that my sister-in-law knows and trusts. I provided the background information needed and pertinent medical history. The clinic I used is D'Arcy Naturals. They ship me the supplements I need and we do a phone consult, as needed, or every three to six months.

Tip: Before buying any supplements or vitamins, make an appointment with an herbalist with experience and credentials. Follow the plan outlined for your particular needs. You need to purchase high-quality products from a reputable shop and take them consistently as directed. Some should be taken with food. Some shouldn't be taken with grapefruit juice (which is not a Ketogenic beverage anyway).

I felt better about ingesting herbs in their natural form whenever possible. For instance, *turmeric* is known to be a cancer fighter. You can buy it in bulk and cook with it or take it in capsule form. Price-wise, it's more cost-effective to buy it in bulk. When added to a glass of water, turmeric is an effective liver cleanser.

Another anti-cancer spice is *cinnamon*. I shake it into coffee and into the blender with smoothies. It's a no-carb wonder and it's good for you.

Fresh *ginger root* is another anti-cancer spice that is easy to use and store. We keep it in the freezer and grate it into the blender to take the edge off bitter greens like kale when making smoothies.

Another anti-cancer spice, *garlic*, adds great flavor and aroma to meals. A garlic press makes it easy to add it to meals. Or, for convenience it can be purchased minced or chopped, ready to serve.

CHAPTER 8

RECOMMENDED SITES AND SUPPORT GROUPS

Medical Support:
www.abta.org
American Brain Tumor Association

www.thebarrow.org
Barrow Neurological Institute
Click on "Research" and "Neuro-Oncology." There's also a link called "Tapping Nutrition to Fight Cancer." Most of the professionals who have helped me are from this amazing organization.

ketogenic-diet-resource.com
This site is the simplest one I've found, and I've been looking for over two years for a direct and easy-to-use guide as a quick reference. I suggest printing out the charts and lists. Laminate them and keep them handy for shopping and meal prep. In addition to the charts, there are also tips and additional helpful information. Included on this site are articles on everything "Keto." I visit it often. There's also a link to a cancer diet ebook. You'll find charts and lists on different sources

of proteins, vegetables, dairy products, nuts and seeds, beverages, acceptable sweeteners, and spices.

Each chart gives caloric content fat grams, carbs in grams, fiber in grams, net carbs and protein in grams. Notice there is no mention of fruit. All fruits except berries are high carb. I only use organic frozen berries. It's easiest to buy the frozen mixed berries of which I'll use 1/4 cup in the Blendtec or as a low carb snack. I prefer frozen to fresh because fresh berries spoil so quickly.

Articles on Dr. Thomas Seyfried (author of *Cancer As A Metabolic Disease* and a pioneer in metabolic therapy for brain cancer): http://articles.mercola.com/sites/articles/archive/2013/06/16/ ketogenic-diet-benefits.aspx

Adrienne C. Scheck's research: www.examiner.com
Low carb ketogenic diet battles brain cancer
by Samantha Chang
June 18, 2014
http://www.examiner.com/article/low-carb-ketogenic-diet-can-manage-brain-cancer-says-scientist-adrienne-scheck

www.perkinelmer.com
For history, explanation, and scientific data of the KD as an adjuvant therapy for brain tumors.

www.examiner.com
Look for a great article called "Low carb Ketogenic diet battles brain cancer, says scientist Adrienne Scheck." Dr. Scheck, as you know by now, has helped me have success with implementing the KD. I'm fortunate to be receiving my care at the BNI and St. Joseph's Hospital, where her research lab is located. I feel like a pioneer!

Foundations:
The Charlie Foundation: www.charliefoundation.org/)
Mathew's Friends: www.matthewsfriends.org/

Reference for a good article on having a spouse with cancer:
www.cancer.voirici.net

Mental/Emotional:
www.berniesiegelmd.com

How to Forgive:
www.wikihow.com/Forgive

Mind Power:
Guidance, tips and advice on the power of the mind, imagination, and the power of thoughts.

www.successconsciousness.com

www.biblegateway.com

www.chrisbeatcancer.com
This is a site I visit almost daily to see the latest survivor stories and Chris's take on anything to do with natural healing. Chris is a regular guy with an amazing story. Just watch a couple of his videos and you'll feel like you know him. He discusses issues related to all kinds of cancers.

www.apple-cider-vinegar-benefits.com

www.wendybanting.com
(Essiac tea)

Recipes and lifestyle support:
www.greensmoothiegirl.com
www.facebook.com/GreenSmoothieGirl

To communicate medical news and updates, we started up a "caring bridge" page. Mine was www.caringbridge.org/mindyelwell (I've since taken it down since my condition has stabilized.)

Some hospitals have their own support sites. Whether a caring bridge or a hospital site, having this hub of communication saves a ton of time by getting your news across to everyone in one click. Without it, we were hard-pressed to make and return phone calls, or answer texts and emails, all exhausting and impossible during the stress of treatment.

Meals on Wheels:
Regional links available online. Our neighborhood is pretty unique in that it's small and people are unusually caring and generous. Someone, I don't know who, got us set up with the meals ministry through our church. The web-site and sign-up was called "Food Tidings."

EPILOGUE

It's been an eventful few years, to the point where I can hardly remember what life was like before cancer. Back in February of 2012, I was a healthy, muscular 135 pounds. The gym was a daily destination and I was ready to embark on my new consulting business. But, of course, you know the story. I try very hard to focus on everything but the negatives, everything that I *can* do and not on what I *can't* do—and what I miss doing. I'm grateful for living beyond that eighteen-month prognosis (October 2013), grateful for seeing my oldest son graduate high school and being able to accompany him to college orientation. I'm looking forward to seeing my other two children go through the same precious rituals.

My most recent test results still show the tumor area to be clear, although balance and weakness is a recurring issue. The doctors believe this could be due to inflammation and the effects of radiation. With over forty treatments, I can't imagine how many healthy brain cells have been zapped, fried, killed. The problem with that, along with irreversible nerve damage, is the dead tissue can't be removed. The body can only do so much to cleanse itself, especially within the brain and skull. I've read that surgery can be an option, in some cases, to remove dead cells if the problem with inflammation becomes severe. Steroids might also an option, but how long can a person take steroids, and at what risk? So many questions…

Here's one last excerpt of medical records I'd like to share. This is from my most recent MRI before the printing of this book, from May 2, 2015, showing an all clear for tumor recurrence.

IMAGING EXAM REPORT

COMPARISON: *03/02/2015 MRI brain an [sic] 08/29/2014 MRI brain*

Technique: Multiplanar multiecho imaging of the brain without and with 10 cc of Multihance intravenous contrast material.

FINDINGS:
Stable postsurgical change related to RIGHT parietal craniotomy. Stable RIGHT corono radiate resection cavity.

Stable FLAIR hyperintensity surrounding the margin of the resection cavity. Stable FLAIR hyperintensity involving the bilateral centrum semiovale and within the bilateral periventricular white matter compared to 03/02/2015. Stable Wallerian degeneration within the RIGHT midbrain and pons. Stable intrinsic T1 hyperintensity adjacent to the RIGHT lateral ventricle white matter. No new or modular enhancement is seen in the region of the resection cavity to indicate recurrent tumor.

There is no restricted diffusion to indicate acute infarct. No acute intracranial hemorrhage. No midline shift or mass effect. Stable ventricular size and configuration. Basal cisterns are patent. Visualized flow voids are unremarkable. Globes and orbits are unremarkable. Paranasal sinuses and mastoid air cells are clear.

IMPRESSION:
1. Stable MRI compared to 03/02/2015. No evidence for tumor recurrence.

* * * * * * * * *

So, while this seems promising, there's no doubt that the long-term effects from forty-five rounds of radiation on the brain, and nerve damage, are irreversible. At this point, I'm on the watch and wait plan. My treatment options include chemotherapy, with Avastin infusions. Anyone that knows about Avastin knows it's very toxic (that's the whole point with chemo, isn't it), with some serious potential side effects, and it's used to help treat a range of cancers, including colorectal cancer, breast cancer, lung cancer, and recurring gliomas. Being on this very expensive drug at this stage of my treatment reminds me that cancer is a force to be reckoned with.

The world is full of powerful forces, rooted in nature, and sometimes unexplainable. If you believe in God, you also believe there's a divine beauty to these forces, especially those that defy logic and man's intervention. Cancer has been around for a very long time and, in spite of all the progress medicine has made over the centuries, it still defies the odds. But there's no beauty in this force of nature, given what it robs of the human body, and the pace of its destruction on even the strongest among us.

I believe in God, and He helps me see beyond cancer, beyond the physical weakness it's causing me—more and more every day. Today, I see what many others don't, because they're still healthy, cancer free. I see what really matters in this world, not material things, not physical beauty, but love and family—my loving husband, and my three beautiful children, growing up before my eyes. I also see my soul; it's my fortress.

In the end, as cancer devours the physical body that is its host, the soul will continue to live, rising up into an even more beautiful world of eternity, beyond cancer's reach. When I get to that world, by my maker's side, I will look down, smile upon my family, and know that while I wait for them to join me, through God's Grace, I did indeed defy and conquer this beast.

"And He said to me, 'My grace is sufficient for you, for My strength is made perfect in weakness.' Therefore most gladly I will rather boast in my infirmities, that the power of Christ may rest upon me."
–2 Corinthians 9

ACKNOWLEDGMENTS

Rich Elwell, my best friend and husband. I know you've suffered with me. Your strength is to be admired. Throughout this journey you've shown a side I'd not known. You jumped in full force and learned all about this disease and its treatments. You were well-prepared and showed great courage. You've protected me along the way from things too scary to discuss. Thank you for holding my head as I cried and for making jokes when I needed to laugh. No matter how many days, weeks, months, or years I have left on this beautiful Earth, I know we'll make every moment count.

Our children, Richie, Angela and Domenic, for understanding my commitment to write this book. We're a great team! Sharing your experiences will help other kids.

Neuro-surgeons Dr. Kris Smith, for the flawless needle biopsy, and Dr. Nader Sanai, for removing my tumor when I thought my options had run out.

Dr. Troy Anderson, Phoenix Neurology and Sleep Medicine, our friend, neighbor and neurologist, for your skill in symptom assessment and for connecting me with Barrow Neurological Institute.

Dr. Shapiro, for your expertise and for teaching me to put things in perspective. Congratulations on your retirement, Rich and I will miss you.

Barrow Neurological Institute nurses, Valerie and Carol, for your compassion and help with the many details of cancer care.

Lee Renda, St. Joseph's dietitian, for helping us understand the Ketogenic diet, and for your support as we learned how to implement it.

Dr. Adrienne Scheck, researcher, whose passion is finding ways to eradicate brain tumors. You renewed our hope for a longer life.

Jasmine Bingham, my co-author and editor, for your patience while I learned the ins and outs of telling my story, and for our many phone conversations and your guidance.

Lorraine Lantz, for connecting me with Balcony 7 Media and Publishing and publisher, Randy Morkved, who agreed to take a chance on a new author and publish my story, as my partner and guide.

Angelique White, for your talent, creativity and encouragement as my photographer.

Sandra Champlain, for lighting the spark in me to begin writing and for your guidance in helping my start be successful.

Erin Davis, for inviting me to writing workshops and for your advice, and Liz Lyons, for guiding me as I learned the writing process.

All of our precious family, friends and neighbors, naming you all would consume an entire chapter. Our family treasures you.

Summit Community Church for the fellowship, friendships, prayers and on-going support.

A NOTE ABOUT THE AUTHORS

Mindy Elwell has a Master's degree in Clinical Psychology from Bridgewater State University in Massachusetts and is a former counselor to troubled teens and their families, who face drug addiction and abuse, as well as those disadvantaged. Her terminal diagnosis of brain cancer set off a courageous battle of survival, leading to a brave surgery to remove the once-inoperable tumor and adopt the Ketogenic Diet, a breakthrough adjuvant therapy for cancer patients, proven to starve cancer cells. She lives in Arizona with her husband and three children.

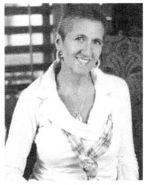

Author Photo:
Angelique White

* * * * * * * * * *

JZ Bingham is a published author and ghost writer, vice president of acquisitions and editor-in-chief of Balcony 7 Media and Publishing and its online magazine, Saucy Jaw. She resides in Pasadena ,California.

Please take the time to leave a review and share your reading experience with others by posting on any or all of the following suggested sites:

Amazon's Defy and Conquer page

Barnes & Noble Defy & Conquer page

Disqus on Publisher's Author Profile page

The author and the production team appreciates all feedback you may share. Please follow Mindy Elwell and Defy & Conquer on these social media sites:

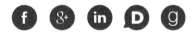

CPSIA information can be obtained at www.ICGtesting.com
Printed in the USA
BVOW11*1054240715

409218BV00001B/1/P